Women and Healthy Aging: Living Productively in Spite of It All

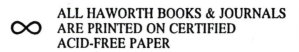

Women
and Healthy Aging:
Living Productively
in Spite of It All

J. Dianne Garner, DSW
Alice A. Young, PhD
Editors

The Haworth Press, Inc.
New York • London • Norwood (Australia)

Women and Healthy Aging: Living Productively in Spite of It All has also been published as *Journal of Women & Aging*, Volume 5, Numbers 3/4 1993.

The development, preparation, and publication of this work has been undertaken with great care. However, the publisher, employees, editors, and agents of The Haworth Press and all imprints of The Haworth Press, Inc., including the Haworth Medical Press and Pharmaceutical Products Press, are not responsible for any errors contained herein or for consequences that may ensue from use of materials or information contained in this work. Opinions expressed by the author(s) are not necessarily those of The Haworth Press, Inc.

The Haworth Press, Inc., 10 Alice Street, Binghamton, NY 13904-1580 USA

Library of Congress Cataloging–in–Publication Data

Women and healthy aging: living productively in spite of it all / J. Dianne Garner, Alice A. Young, editors.
    p.   cm.
    "Has also been published as Journal of women & aging, volume 5, numbers 3/4 1993"–T.p. verso
    Includes bibliographical references and index.
    ISBN 1-56023-049-5 (hpp : alk. paper).–ISBN 1-56024-509-3 (alk. paper)
    1. Aged women–Diseases. 2. Adjustment (Psychology) in old age. 3. Aged women–Health and hygiene. 4. Aged women–Mental health. 5. Self-actualization (Psychology) in old age. 6. Aged women–Medical care–United States. I. Garner, J. Dianne. II. Young, Alice Adam.
    [DNLM: 1. Aging–physiology. 2. Women's Health. 3. Women's Health Services–United States. 4. Quality of Life. WT 104 W872 1993]
RA564.85.W625 1993
362.1'9897'0082–dc20
DNLM/DLC   93-40755
for Library of Congress   CIP

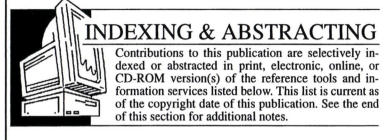

INDEXING & ABSTRACTING

Contributions to this publication are selectively indexed or abstracted in print, electronic, online, or CD-ROM version(s) of the reference tools and information services listed below. This list is current as of the copyright date of this publication. See the end of this section for additional notes.

- *Abstracts in Anthropology*, Baywood Publishing Company, 26 Austin Avenue, P.O. Box 337, Amityville, NY 11701

- *Abstracts in Social Gerontology: Current Literature on Aging*, National Council on the Aging, Library, 409 Third Street SW, 2nd Floor, Washington, DC 20024

- *Abstracts of Research in Pastoral Care & Counseling*, Loyola College, 7135 Minstrel Way, Suite 101, Columbia, MD 21045

- *Academic Index (on-line)*, Information Access Company, 362 Lakeside Drive, Foster City, CA 94404

- *Ageline Database*, American Association of Retired Persons, 601 E Street NW, Washington DC 20049

- *Behavioral Medicine Abstracts*, The Society of Behavioral Medicine, 103 South Adams Street, Rockville, MD 20850

- *Cambridge Scientific Abstracts*, *Risk Abstracts*, Cambridge Information Group, 7200 Wisconsin Avenue #601, Bethesda, MD 20814

- *Feminist Periodicals: A Current Listing of Contents*, Women's Studies Librarian-at-Large, 728 State Street, 430 Memorial Library, Madison, WI 53706

- *Guide to Social Science & Religion in Periodical Literature*, National Periodical Library, P.O. Box 3278, Clearwater, FL 34630

(continued)

- *Human Resources Abstracts*, Sage Publications, Inc., 2455 Teller Road, Newbury Park, CA 91320

- *Index to Periodical Articles Related to Law*, University of Texas, 727 East 26th Street, Austin, TX 78705

- *Inventory of Marriage and Family Literature (online and hard copy)*, National Council on Family Relations, 3989 Central Avenue NE, Suite 550, Minneapolis, MN 55421

- *Mental Health Abstracts (online through DIALOG)*, IFI/Plenum Data Company, 3202 Kirkwood Highway, Wilmington, DE 19808

- *Periodical Abstracts, Research 2*, UMI Data Courier, P.O. Box 32770, Louisville, KY 40232-2770

- *SilverPlatter Information, Inc.* **"CD-ROM/online,"** Information Resources Group, 101 West Walnut Street, Suite 200, Pasadena, CA 91103

- *Social Planning/Policy & Development Abstracts (SOPODA)*, Sociological Abstracts, Inc., P.O. Box 22206, San Diego, CA 92192-0206

- *Social Work Research & Abstracts*, National Association of Social Workers, 750 First Street NW, 8th Floor, Washington, DC 20002

- *Sociological Abstracts (SA)*, Sociological Abstracts, Inc., P.O. Box 22206, San Diego, CA 92192-0206

- *Studies on Women Abstracts*, Carfax Publishing Company, P.O. Box 25, Abingdon, Oxfordshire OX14 3UE, United Kingdom

- *Women Studies Abstracts,* Rush Publishing Company, P.O. Box 1, Rush, NY 14543

- *Women's Studies Index (indexed comprehensively),* G.K. Hall & Co., 866 Third Avenue, New York, NY 10022

SPECIAL BIBLIOGRAPHIC NOTES

related to indexing, abstracting, and library access services

☐ indexing/abstracting services in this list will also cover material in the "separate" that is co-published simultaneously with Haworth's special thematic journal issue or DocuSerial. Indexing/abstracting usually covers material at the article/chapter level.

☐ monographic co-editions are intended for either non-subscribers or libraries which intend to purchase a second copy for their circulating collections.

☐ monographic co-editions are reported to all jobbers/wholesalers/approval plans. The source journal is listed as the "series" to assist the prevention of duplicate purchasing in the same manner utilized for books-in-series.

☐ to facilitate user/access services all indexing/abstracting services are encouraged to utilize the co-indexing entry note indicated at the bottom of the first page of each article/chapter/contribution.

☐ this is intended to assist a library user of any reference tool (whether print, electronic, online, or CD-ROM) to locate the monographic version if the library has purchased this version but not a subscription to the source journal.

☐ individual articles/chapters in any Haworth publication are also available through the Haworth Document Delivery Services (HDDS).

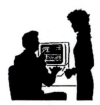

Women and Healthy Aging: Living Productively in Spite of It All

CONTENTS

ABOUT THE EDITORS

J. Dianne Garner, DSW, is currently Professor and Chair of the Department of Social Work at Washburn University, Topeka, KS, and Chair of the Washburn University Center on Aging. Dr. Garner was previously the Director of Social Work at Cedars-Sinai Medical Center in Los Angeles as well as on the faculty at California State University at Long Beach. A long-time member of the National Association of Social Workers, she has served as National Second Vice-President for two years as well as Regional Representative, President of the Arkansas Chapter, and Chair of the National Committee on Women's Issues. She is a co-editor of the book *Women as They Age: Challenge, Opportunity and Triumph* (The Haworth Press, Inc., 1989), and author of several journal articles, books, and numerous papers presented at national, state, and local meetings on the elderly. Dr. Garner has been listed in the *Who's Who Among Human Services Professionals*, Third Edition, 1992-93 and the *Who's Who of Women Executives* listing in 1989-90.

Alice A. Young, PhD, is Professor and Dean of the School of Nursing at Washburn University in Topeka, KS, where she has been responsible for the development and administration of the nursing program since its inception in 1974. Previously, she taught nursing at New York University, The College of St. Catherine, and Catholic University. Dr. Young has been President of the Kansas State Nurses Association and of Hospice, Inc., of Topeka. She has served on the Editorial Board of *Kansas Nurse* and is the author of several journal articles and numerous paper presentations at national, state, and local conferences.

Introduction

J. Dianne Garner, DSW
Alice A. Young, PhD

American women are enjoying dramatic increases in longevity: In the 1990s the average lifespan for women will surpass the age of 80. Women currently make up about two-thirds of people over 85 and for every 100 women over the age of 85, there are only 36 men (Task Force for Aging Research Funding [TFARF] 1992). While women over 65 tend to report better overall health than do men in the same age group (Special Committee on Aging, United States Senate, 1990), as a result of longevity, women are more prone to chronic illnesses and conditions associated with aging. Arthritis, cardiovascular diseases, stroke, breast cancer and osteoporosis disproportionately affect older women. Among women, approximately 94 percent of heart attacks and 80 percent of breast cancers occur post menopause. More than 4 million women age 65 and over are moderately to severely disabled as a result of disease and age-related changes, representing about two-thirds of all disabled elderly (TFARF, 1992).

While disease and age-related changes pose significant challenges to older women, the picture is not as bleak as it may seem. Countless older women overcome the adversity of disease and physical changes daily, continuing to live highly productive lives and making significant contributions to families, friends and/or communities. Irene Burnside, our lead author in this work, is a prime example of an older woman who continues to live produc-

[Haworth co-indexing entry note]: "Introduction." Garner, J. Dianne, and Alice A. Young. Co-published simultaneously in the *Journal of Women & Aging* (The Haworth Press, Inc.) Vol. 5, No. 3/4, 1993, pp. 1-6; and: *Women and Healthy Aging: Living Productively in Spite of It All* (ed: J. Dianne Garner, and Alice A. Young), The Haworth Press, Inc., 1993, pp. 1-6. Multiple copies of this article/chapter may be purchased from The Haworth Document Delivery Center [1-800-3-HAWORTH; 9:00 a.m.-5:00 p.m. (EST)].

tively with adversity. Since her formal "retirement" and appointment as Professor Emerita at San Jose State University, Irene has completed her Ph.D. in nursing, trotted all over the world lecturing and doing research, published numerous articles, book chapters and complete books and continues to teach, currently as a visiting professor at the University of North Carolina at Greensboro. Oh yes, in between all her activities, she managed to sandwich intermittent chemotherapy and radiation treatments for cancer. It is no accident that Irene was asked to lead us in our efforts. Another fine example of a feisty older woman is Maggie Kuhn, illustrious leader of the Gray Panthers. Maggie came literally shuffling through Kansas a few years ago. Undaunted and unstopped by her own advanced arthritis, she called upon us to recognize the power of older women and to get up off our backsides and make a difference in our communities and nation.

Personally, and in our years as a hospital social worker and a nurse, respectively, we have seen many older women who remained productive and active in spite of illnesses and the changes associated with aging. The old woman, at Ohio State University Hospital who, in 1970, had had metastatic cancer for nineteen years, lived alone in her own home, and episodically came in for treatment. She had hobbies, friends and continued to do community volunteer work. None of her many physicians understood how she was still alive. Her often repeated statement to them as they puzzled over the miracle of her life was "I'm too busy to die." Wilma Maud Roebuck, living in central Arkansas, and in her 90s plagued by deteriorating retinas, continued her love of gardening. Occasionally, she would mistakenly pull a flower rather than a weed. When chastised by her daughter, "Mother you can't see well enough to do this," she was overheard to reply, "It's my garden and I'll tend to it until I decide I can't." Even when osteoporotic fractures began to occur, she stubbornly maintained her own residence. Until her death at the age of 96, she continued to be the clearinghouse for family news. "Now, most of the time, we don't even know what's going on with our brother or sisters, their children or grandchildren." Donna Love, in her 70th year began experiencing pain in her shoulder after a strenuous round of golf. Shortly thereafter, she found herself in the emergency room of a local hospital and subsequently had quintuple bypasses. Today, she is Professor Emerita at Washburn University, Field Coordinator of the social work program and continues to play golf. Martha Rogers, Professor Emerita at New York University, internationally known theorist, educator and scholar in the field of Nursing, in her 79th year is still traveling the world over lecturing, consulting and writing about the Science of Unitary Human Beings. Despite grave respiratory difficulties and frail body structure, she is a woman of iron who views aging as an "evolutionary emergent." Her attitude in life is summed up in her comment during a recent professional interview: "My god, what a fantastic time to be alive!" These women, like Irene and Maggie, are (or were) more lively than most "healthy" people among us. The quality of their lives and their large and small contributions attest to the position that "health" among women in the later years is not necessarily related to the absence of disease or impairments but rather to their determination, spirit and ability to continue to function, overcoming or living with adversity every step of the way and having a vision beyond the immediate, with agendas of work yet to be done.

While not a laundry list of diseases, impairments or changes which impact the lives of older women, we have selected those which appear to affect significant numbers of older women for presentation and exploration in this work. Alzheimer's Disease, the most common form of dementia, affects approximately 4 million older Americans, the majority of whom are women. Various forms of arthritis affect an estimated 37 million Americans, and about half of all Americans over the age of 65 have arthritis. In the United States, 60 percent of all cancers occur in people 65 or older. In fact, age is the single greatest risk factor for cancer. About half of all cases of breast, uterine and ovarian cancer occur in women age 65 and older. Heart attack is the number one killer of older American women, claiming almost three times as many lives as breast cancer and lung cancer combined. At older ages, women who have heart attacks are twice as likely as men to die from them within a few weeks. Approximately half of all diabetics are over the age of 55 and more than 150,000 deaths per year are caused by diabetes and its complications. Osteoporosis affects 20 million women in the U.S. and leads to approximately 1.5 million fractures per year. Vision and hearing impairments, while not diseases, affect the quality of life and threaten the independence of millions of older women (TFARF, 1992).

Since many diseases, including breast cancer, heart attack and osteoporosis are especially influenced by the loss of estrogen after menopause, the second selection of this work is devoted to exploring the effects of menopause. Authors with expertise about the selected disease categories then present an overview of the specific disease, treatment options and strategies for living productively with the respective illness or changes.

The literature is scarce regarding the factors that influence productive, "healthy" living among women in their later years. Nonetheless, a combination of what few studies exist and our own observations as professionals indicate that there are commonalities among the Irene Burnsides and Maggie Kuhns of the world. Strong coping mechanisms, continued activities and involvements, strong human supports in terms of families and/or friends, a sense of humor and the ability to compartmentalize or deny, but not to the extent of endangering themselves seem to be dominant among the characteristics of older women who keep right on leaping over multiple obstacles. They refuse to become their diseases even though the medical system focuses almost exclusively on their diseases. Those who do well seem to know that they are more than the ailments which plague them. In short, there seems to be a very real connection between the human spirit and the ability to live productively with, and overcome the residuals of, illnesses. Conversely, the business of living productively appears to have very real positive effects on the course of diseases and ultimate outcomes.

Another factor is the presence in communities of a variety of services which foster independence and assist older women in making the most of their many remaining assets. As professionals, we know that, when women live long enough, some parts are going to wear out and some diseases will inevitably occur. The automobile with 150,000 miles on it generally has more dents, old age spots and worn parts than the automobile with 15,000 miles on it. We could argue, however, that the old car is, in fact, the better car, having proven itself over and over again. And if that car is old enough we call it an antique, provide it with the necessary parts to keep it running no matter how slowly, value it highly and show it off with great pride. We, unfortunately, do not seem to have the same attitudes toward age and durability in people. With old women we tend to see only the age spots and the worn parts which often defy our skills as "healers." As a consequence availability of services which stress maintenance and independence continue to lag far behind the availability of services which have been traditionally "curative" in nature.

In this society which for so long has stressed "cure" as the appropriate role of health care professionals, what are we to do with the legions of older women whose "cures" may not be possible? How can we help them prevent or slow the occurrence of changes or diseases? And when prevention or cure is not possible, how do we assist them in living productive, meaningful lives? Some suggestions and answers to those questions are explored in each work on specific diseases. It is our hope that our readers will be able to adapt what is here to their own practices and will begin to explore and publish other successful strategies for increasing "healthy," productive aging among older women.

Unfortunately, women, particularly older women, have tended to be discriminated against by our health care system in a number of ways. As a result of that discrimination, there is a move afoot in a segment of the medical community to establish a new medical specialty devoted to women's health. "Its practitioners would be trained in everything from managing menopause to spotting abuse, with a focus on the growing body of research on how diseases and drugs act differently in women than men" (Lewin, 1992, p. C-3). We have, therefore, chosen to devote two essays in this work to an exploration of discrimination against older women and to public policies which affect older women.

As editors and authors moved through the process of creating this work, there were many questions which repeatedly surfaced. Where is the research which systematically studies those older women who do so very well with the changes and diseases which, in fact, occur among women as they age? Do we not, as professionals, have a responsibility to do more than dispense medication, remove diseased tissue and otherwise treat illnesses? Should we not also be helping older women commit to life, encouraging them to be active, helping them find support groups and networks? Should we not be working with families and our own colleagues to treat older women as worthwhile, contributing human beings who have a right to make their own decisions? And finally, do we not have a responsibility to remind ourselves of the humanity of older women who, incidentally happen to have some illnesses or age-related changes? There is a sense among the authors here that as long as we treat older women as diseases rather than as capable functioning people, we are contributing to their sense of no longer having worth or ability and to the subsequent depressions that so frequently accompany medical diagnoses and age-related changes. So let us approach these pages with the realization that the medical information contained herein is important, but no more so than the strategies which assist aging women in living productive, healthy lives. Let us also remember that it is the older women themselves who can teach us so very much about the business of overcoming adversity.

REFERENCES

Lewin, T. (1992) Women fight to overcome male bias in medicine. *San Diego Union-Tribune*, November 17, p. C-3.

Special Committee on Aging, United States Senate (1991) *Developments in aging: 1990, Volume 1*, Washington D.C.: U.S. Government Printing Office.

Task Force for Aging Research Funding (1992) *Independence for older Americans: Real answers to health & aging*, Washington D.C.: Alliance for Aging Research.

Adaptations

Older women will hack new roles
with a teaspoon out of permafrost.
When you compliment their strength,
they will offer you a spoonful.
They will create welcoming homes
from scotch tape and garage sales.
When you sink into the comfort,
they will say "anyone can do it."
They will share lifesaving wisdom
sending no bill for their services
and thank you for listening.

–Ruth Harriet Jacobs, PhD

Ruth Harriet Jacobs is Researcher, Wellesley College Center for Research on Women, Wellesley, MA 02181.

[Haworth co-indexing entry note]: "Adaptations." Jacobs, Ruth Harriet. Co-published simultaneously in the *Journal of Women & Aging* (The Haworth Press, Inc.) Vol. 5, No. 3/4, 1993, p. 7; and: *Women and Healthy Aging: Living Productively in Spite of It All* (ed: J. Dianne Garner, and Alice A. Young), The Haworth Press, Inc., 1993, p. 7. Multiple copies of this article/chapter may be purchased from The Haworth Document Delivery Center [1-800-3-HAWORTH; 9:00 a.m.-5:00 p.m. (EST)].

Healthy Older Women–
In Spite of It All

Irene Burnside, PhD, RN, FAAN

SUMMARY. Health in older women in this discussion is considered from four perspectives of fitness: (a) physical, (b) intellectual, (c) social and (d) purpose. The important point is that it is not health, per se, which is so crucial in women's later lives, but rather their attitudes and their coping strategies to meet new situations, losses and crises. In addition, the responses of others, including professionals, are important in enabling older women to live productive lives in spite of adversity. Examples of positive models of women growing old with varying degrees of health problems are provided.

Age seldom arrives smoothly or quickly. It's more a series of jerks.

—J. Rhys (1975)

The term "well elderly" is probably a euphemism since many older people do have varying degrees of health-related problems. The popular, often quoted World Health Organization's definition of health "a state of complete physical, mental and social well-being and not merely the absence of disease or infirmity" (WHO; as cited

---

Irene Burnside is Visiting Professor, School of Nursing, University of North Carolina at Greensboro. Address correspondence to: 11509 Fury Lane #7, El Cajon, CA 92019.

[Haworth co-indexing entry note]: "Healthy Older Women–In Spite of It All." Burnside, Irene. Co-published simultaneously in the *Journal of Women & Aging* (The Haworth Press, Inc.) Vol. 5, No. 3/4, 1993, pp. 9-24; and: *Women and Healthy Aging: Living Productively in Spite of It All* (ed: J. Dianne Garner, and Alice A. Young), The Haworth Press, Inc., 1993, pp. 9-24. Multiple copies of this article/chapter may be purchased from The Haworth Document Delivery Center [1-800-3-HAWORTH; 9:00 a.m.-5:00 p.m. (EST)].

in Birren and Zarit, 1985, p. 5) rarely applies to the older age cohorts. However, if one views it from a conceptual perspective, it is especially relevant to defining the health of the elderly (Schroot, 1988). People of any age may have some degree of disease, but if they do not "act" ill, they will describe themselves as being healthy (Birren & Zarit, 1985, p. 5). It is possible that others may view older persons as healthy if they do not take on the sick role. As early as 1959, the World Health Organization specifically defined health in older persons as best measured "in function . . . degree of fitness rather than extent of pathology may be used as a measure of the amount of services the aged will require from the community" (WHO; as cited in Miller, 1990, p. 61).

It is also important to make a distinction between the two terms "disease" and "illness" when describing the health of older people. While disease is "a condition of the living animal or plant body of one of its parts that impairs the performance of a vital function" *(Webster's Ninth New Collegiate Dictionary*, 1988), illness refers to the presence of a specific disease, but more than that, it includes the person's perceptions and behaviors in response to the disease, as well as the impact of the disease on the person's psychosocial environment (Ouslander & Beck, 1982). Miller (1990) noted that typical definitions of illness related by older people involved an inability to sleep, eat, walk or be cured. In addition, she cites an older woman, who was wheelchair-bound due to severe arthritis, who defined health as "being helpful to others" (p. 62).

Perhaps, it is best for professionals to focus on the positive aspects in older women and to emphasize fitness and the individual's response to illness. Only then will we begin to recognize what factors contribute to healthy and productive aging among older women–in spite of it all.

> In the evening there are stars that cannot be seen in the daytime. There really are.
>
> –A.D. Carlson, 1977, p. 36

DEMOGRAPHICS

It is common knowledge today that women live longer than men. The life expectancy at birth for a woman in 1984 was 78.2 years compared with a man's life expectancy of 71.2 years, which means the vast majority of the oldest old will be women (Bould, Sanborn & Reif, 1989). By the time women reach the age of 85 or older, there are 220 women to every 100 men. Therefore, "Does one need to ask if demography shapes, in part, the destiny of older women?" (Mercer & Garner, 1989, p. 17).

RESEARCH

Most studies have been on men so we do not have the needed data base for health in older women. Matteson and McConnell (1988) noted the paucity of research on the aging of women in two areas: the response of women to their own retirement and research on menopause from both the feminist and health perspective. However, one need only to scour the literature to uncover the scarcity of research on aging women across the spectrum. Nevertheless, "as a personal experience, old age is as much a woman's concern as a man's–even more so, indeed, since women live longer. But when there is speculation upon the subject, it is considered primarily in terms of men" (de Beauvoir, 1972, p. 89).

Major influences on health and the health care of older women have been noted by Matteson and McConnell (1988), including the negative influences of lower economic status of older women on their health and the lack of research on women and the aging process which results in few norms for women in advanced age. The result of the latter is that older women risk not having treatment based on solid research. However, it appears that research neglect may be ending with federal recommendations now placing a national priority on women's health and there is now a national Office of Research on Women's Health (U.S. Public Health Service, 1991/1992).

In a recent lead article in the *Wall Street Journal*, McCarthy (1992) discusses the plight of elders in detail. "For three decades, the U.S. has essentially defined aging as a medical problem, for which nursing homes have been the answer" (p. 1). Women are the predominant residents in nursing homes, and most of them are doomed to environments that dehumanize them, often ignore their psychosocial needs and do not offer the privacy and independence so many of them crave.

An assisted living residence, Rackleff House, in Oregon is described. A woman who is 92 came there and missed playing the organ she had at home. Rackleff paid for a used organ that is in the dining room, and she plays every day prior to lunch. Note that the woman has had a brain aneurysm and has a bad heart.

All but two of the examples cited in the article pertain to women. Another example given is of a woman who has Alzheimer's disease. She loves to linger by the copy machine in the office at Rackleff. "She had been a bookkeeper most of her working life, and, in her mental confusion, finds the office bustle comforting. Rackleff staffers work around her" (p. 1).

It is not the purpose of this discussion to focus on the environments of elderly women, but it is important for health professionals to realize how profoundly all of us are affected by the environment in which we must live, especially if it is one we did not choose, would never have chosen and know that we will not be able to leave.

CATEGORIES OF FITNESS

According to Butler (1991), there are four important categories of fitness which are essential to maintain as one ages. The first is, of course, physical fitness. The second is intellectual fitness, the third is social fitness and the last category is purpose fitness. These four categories provide a useful framework for professionals working with older women. While it is true that an older woman may not excel in fitness in all four of the areas, the women who serve as our role models for successful aging, in spite of health problems, seem to attain an overall fitness.

> The changes that take place as we get older occur so gradually that they largely escape our notice.
>
> –O. Knopf, 1975, p. 27

Physical Fitness

Physical fitness includes bodily strength, resilience and agility attained by appropriate exercise (Butler, 1991). That does not mean those who are physically fit have been spared disease. In fact, if one really studies some of the women who cope with arthritis, hypertension or cancer, for example, one observes that health has taken on a new (or different) meaning for them. Subsequent sections of this work will address the impact of various diseases on older women with strategies for remaining productive in spite of the presence of disease.

Women with chronic diseases often work assiduously at improving their health status by being "good patients," including following treatment regimens. They also learn to quickly respond to signals from their aging bodies. They do not sign up for high-impact aerobics knowing their aging, arthritic knees won't respond favorably to Step Classes. Awareness of their limitations is another attribute of these women. What seems most healthy in these older women is their healthy attitude, plus an amazing agility to cope, including substituting other activities for those which are no longer doable and/or participating in the same activities but learning to do them in a different manner. Even those who are old-old or seem very frail can surprise us with their abilities. During a reminiscence therapy group, my co-leader and I were being very supportive of a ninety-plus year old, frail woman who had had the book of losses thrown at her. We were not sure she would even accept the group experience; however, she stayed with the group. Initially, she came in a wheelchair. Then, each session, one of us began going to her room and walking with her to meetings. What surprised us was how quickly she became motivated and how her ambulation improved even during the few weeks of the group experience.

Women in their 80s and 90s may not be common sights in the local health club, but many are still gardening and can even be found up on ladders cleaning windows or pruning shrubs. Many of them wear the work ethic well and wear it with pride. Gordon (1989) makes the important point that "Women are often more active if they have been at home for many years since raising children and housekeeping require more physical effort than working in an office." For older women who do not have a car, walking is a must. A septuagenarian acquaintance of mine encouraged me to walk with her because she said "it will get all those perkomorphs going"–her way of saying how important is the role of endorphins.

Not only does laughter provide a medicine all its own to the person laughing, it also creates a mood, a certain ambiance that is welcomed by caregivers.

Couch potatoes are not restricted to the younger generation and one cannot deny the role television plays in the lives of some older women as they design their daily schedules around the soap operas. Would that they would heed Rossman's (1988) advice that exercise is "a major antidote to the aging process" (p. 229). Roberto, in a later section of this publication, gives an excellent example of the importance of physical exercise in osteoporosis. She writes about "consistent participation in weight-bearing activities" to both maximize and maintain bone mass in older women.

We are reminded "that the realities of aging cannot necessarily be avoided; however, quality of life can be maintained by doing things differently, in spite of obstacles" (Garner, personal letter, 1992). She gives a powerful example of overcoming physical handicaps:

> I think of my grandmother. When in her 90's, her vision was severely compromised by deteriorating retinas and her hands were deformed by arthritis. She had oil painted all her life. But when her buildings began to lean and facial features blurred, she simply switched to modern art. She died at 96, still living in her own home in the hills of central Arkansas . . . She bowed out having her traditional 5:00 a.m. cup of coffee.

This superb example of adaptive artistic abilities leads us into the next category, maintaining intellectual functioning.

Intellectual Fitness

One prominent researcher in gerontology states that "The evidence suggests that most older adults have not grown old sick, poor and lonely. Indeed, they are more concerned with opportunities for learning and experimenting with life than the young are prepared to believe" (Birren, 1978, p. 206). But some families have difficulty because they are stuck in the "old dog cannot learn new tricks" rut. In the area where I live, the adult education classes do a booming business. And nowhere is that more apparent than in the computer classes. These classes are the only ones for which one must pre-register. Older people bring their folding chairs at 5:00 a.m. to await the 7:30 opening of the registration office. In addition, older women I have talked to have praised the benefits of "Elder Hostel" programs which provide intellectual stimulation, travel opportunities and socialization as well–all rolled into one package.

Vischer (1967) stated that "Old age has been defined as the period of life in which we experience fewer and fewer things for the first time and more and more things for the last time. The ability to receive new and original impressions as new and original, the ability to be surprised by life, is perhaps a criterion of psycho-spiritual health in aging persons." Classes at all levels, whether credit or non-credit, help the older woman to generate "new and original impressions."

In older women, stress may have some negative functional consequences on intellectual abilities. A study of older women by Sands (1981-82) found that high levels of stress did contribute to a decline in intellectual functioning. In the same study, a relationship was identified between intellectual functioning and specific stressful events. For example, changes in personal health or the health of a family member were positively correlated with declines in intellectual functioning.

Work and intellectual stimulation can certainly help in coping with the stress caused by illnesses in later life. I decided to revise a book during the time I had radiation therapy for cancer. Because the technicians were rarely on schedule, I took manuscripts with me to the clinic to proofread as I sat. One day the oncologist asked me what I was doing. When I told her, she asked to see what I was proofreading. She apparently relayed this information to the nurses who worked there. Proofreading not only kept my mind occupied and functioning, in spite of cancer and cancer treatment, it provided a topic for future conversations. Those exchanges with the nurses were much different from the typical conversations in medical treatment centers which generally focus almost exclusively on the illness and can increase the stress of the person coping with cancer. It is not easy to accept disease, but old age may not be easy to accept either.

". . . identifying oneself as old is not easy. No wonder our ambition tends to be to 'stay young' rather than to *become* the best possible old person. To become the 'best possible' elder is a very difficult, highly creative undertaking and should be so regarded by both the old person and those around . . . " her.

–A. D. Carlson, 1977, p. 36

Social Fitness

The social fitness category is defined as needing to accomplish "forming and maintaining significant personal relationships that may be called upon in good times and in bad" (Butler, 1991, p. vii). There are a variety of ways older women work on social fitness. Some are very active in their churches; others are enrolled in the classes described earlier and acquire new friendships in the classroom. Other women volunteer many hours to charitable work and maintain their social fitness because they feel they are making a contribution and that they are needed.

Groups should always be considered as a means of helping older women acquire and/or maintain social fitness (Burnside, 1989; 1986). Potential groups need to be considered in all settings: low cost housing and affluent retirement homes, as well as nursing homes and day care programs. Birren and Deutchman (1991) note that their guided autobiography groups are not designed as formal therapy. However, they are therapeutic because the members develop friendships with other group members.

Reminiscence and Social Fitness

Reminiscence therapy is one strategy to enhance social fitness for older women and is implemented by a variety of health professionals. Reminiscence therapy may be introduced in a dyad situation, for example, in a health assessment or intake interview, or it may be implemented as a group modality (Burnside, in press). The intervention may be used in a variety of settings, and older women are found in any setting that provides health care or assisted living. Hamilton (1992) reminds us that "Patients who are eager to reminisce need only encouragement . . . in order to elicit a stream of thought and conversation about the past" (p. 296). The same author advises the health care worker to begin "where the patient is emotionally and proceed sensibly. A judgmental attitude, poor timing, inappropriate interpretations or confrontations will be met with defenses such as anger or denial" (p. 297). I did not proceed sensibly with one group. A very frail and very old woman in my first group in the late 1960s zeroed in on my anxiety as a new group leader. I was asking many questions to get something started in the group. Finally this alert woman across from me in her chirpy, no-nonsense manner asked, "Why are you being so crusty?" Since that feedback, I have been a lot less crusty in all group meetings with older people. One of the powerful effects of reminiscence in a group for the older woman is the sense of connectedness (Burnside, 1990). Women with few remaining families or peers can find a connection with other women when they become a part of an ongoing group. In this study (Burnside, 1990) of community-based women, other results were reported in the qualitative component of the study: self-affirmation, others-affirmation and reflection. The most important meaning for the group experience for the elderly women reminiscers was being able to compare their lives to the lives of other women in the group followed by "fellowship" and "enjoyment."

Reminiscence therapy also provides the health care professional with information on how the older woman has coped in the past with crises and health-related problems. Such knowledge may be a predictor of what the health care professional can expect of the client in the present situation.

Genealogy and Social Fitness

The genealogical activities of older women could fit under both the intellectual and social fitness categories. It requires sleuthing ability to track down ancestors and there has been increased interest observed in older women in their interest in leaving legacies to relatives in the form of autobiographies (Birren & Deutchman, 1991), journals (Sarton, 1973; 1980; 1984; Scott-Maxwell, 1969; Vining, 1978), or tracing the family history. Last year I attended a genealogy class in a local senior center. The class was comprised of 90 percent women and about 10 percent men; only a couple of students were not in the stage of later life. The intensity and perseverance with which these women pursued their roots was amazing. The poignant stories told in class about ancestors and how they found out about them were as intriguing as those one hears in a reminiscence therapy group. Recently there have been a number of grandmother (and grandfather) books designed to facilitate the recall of memories for older adults.

The social fitness pattern selected by an older woman may not meet the approval of her family or peers. De Beauvoir (1972) points out that "for women in particular the last age is liberation" (p. 488). A popular French movie that we used during the 1970s for teaching is entitled "The Shameless Old Lady." It is a fine example of a truly liberated older woman. At the age of 72 she is left a widow. Her family is aghast as she indulges herself in the things that she now desires. She had previously behaved according to expected standards. She gives those up. She rides in a carriage, goes out to eat and goes to visit a cobbler, who is of a different social class. Her children could not understand her new quest for life. One lovely scene captures the essence of the film and her liberation. The "shameful old lady" sits alone on the bank of a river looking out on moon-decorated water. She pulls the hair pins out of her bun and the winds of the night blow through her long, thinning, gray hair.

> The intoxicating feeling of freedom repays you a thousand times for any loneliness you may have endured–The other compensation is the calm that often comes with age.
>
> –J. Rhys, 1975

We have not emphasized enough the importance of relationships between grandmothers and grandchildren in maintaining social fitness. During the time in my life when I was trying to adjust to and accept multiple diagnoses, I found that the grandchildren brought something very special to me. When you can collapse cancer into a simple "owie," it becomes less complicated and complex to be sure. Children's perceptions also help us with our own ability to generate "new and original" impressions because they are the masters of that ability.

Though, perhaps, not a part of social fitness, per se, an unexpected source of frustration and stress that I did not know how to deal with was the rumor that I had died. I wrote a colleague for a copy of an article she had written and it came back with a poignant note stating how glad she was to get my letter because she had heard that I was dead. I do not believe Miss Manners has written about how to respond to such comments. I often wonder how others have dealt with this occurrence post illness. My own solution was to go to every conference and meeting and be very visible to quell the rumor and to demonstrate a bit of physical, intellectual, social and purpose fitness.

Purpose Fitness

"Purpose fitness means having feelings of self-esteem and control over one's life" (Butler, 1990, p. vii). The "shameless old woman," much to her family's consternation, had taken control of her life. She found new and different purposes for her last years.

There are many mechanisms for maintaining self-esteem and control over one's life through purpose. Whether it be knowing that we must provide food and love to a pet, that others, less fortunate than ourselves, depend on our formal and informal volunteer activities or that we continue to make contributions through paid work, having purpose is essential for productive, healthy living at all stages of life and no less so in the later years.

Family members who are determined to call all the shots certainly make it difficult for older women to maintain purpose fitness. One of the most poignant examples of not having control in a social situation occurred at a wedding I attended many years ago. I sat with the bride's grandmother and her peers. They were enjoying the beautiful wedding–all but the music. The grandmother had finished a glass of champagne and the caterer came with a tray. Just as she reached out to take a glass, a hand intercepted it and placed it back on the tray. Her granddaughter had been walking by the table, and in a loud voice, she sternly said, "No, grandma, you have had enough already." The look on the old woman's face said it all. With those few words, her joy and self-esteem withered leaving behind a noticeably quieter and older woman.

HUMANIZATION OF THE OLDER WOMAN

Perhaps we could begin the humanization of the older woman in such a simple way as just described–not to make decisions for her, especially in front of others. It is so common that relatives feel that they must speak for older women and make their decisions, even though they have never been asked for advice. Dorothy Moses was one of the pioneers in gerontological nursing. But what she taught me in the classroom was not as powerful as what she taught me at her mother's bedside in a nursing home one day. After a class, we stopped to see her mother. Her mother was bedridden and frail. When Dorothy asked if there was anything she could do, her mother replied that she wanted a box of cards sorted. It was high on the shelf in her closet. I sat in a corner and watched the interaction. Each card was examined and then the decision made whether to save it or to toss it out. At no point did Dorothy make any suggestions. Only when her mother faltered a bit about a name did Dorothy remind her who the sender was. That exercise in restraint, patience and decision-making stays in my mind.

SELF-ESTEEM

Self esteem is an important component of purpose fitness. It should also be noted that self-esteem is closely associated with both physical health and functional abilities. Self-esteem is diminished at times of illness. Interventions should be directed toward helping the older person improve functional abilities to help enhance their self-esteem (Miller, 1990).

Those of us who have been hospitalized have countless stories to tell about the put-downs, the impatient and abrupt personnel and what such actions do to one's self-esteem. These behaviors of professionals in health care may give us some clues to how they perceive older women. Recently a woman in her mid-sixties was in the emergency room of a hospital. She had been injured while traveling and was highly stressed. However, she did not lose her sense of humor when she heard a very young resident out in the hall yell to the nurse, "Where is the chart on that little old lady who was assaulted?" It was the first time she had ever been designated a "little old lady." One is reminded of Simon de Beauvoir's line, "If I did not keep telling myself my age over and over again, I am sure I should scarcely be aware of it" (p. 295). Perhaps we should add, "and if others did not keep reminding me" to de Beauvoir's line.

In addition to the negative implications of being designated "the little old lady" is the depersonalization of being rendered nameless and its resulting assault to self-esteem. All too often, as professionals, we refer to hospitalized patients as room 712, bed 1 or the gall bladder in room 309. We barge into their temporary residences, on which they are paying a rather substantial rent, without knocking. We perform our tasks without conversation or with minimal conversation which only concerns their dysfunctions or illnesses. Many times we do not even make eye contact. Nowhere are these behaviors more obvious than with the old who have the audacity not to be "curable."

It is imperative that professionals recognize that our behavior can be curative, if not to the disease, to the spirit and to the self-esteem of the older women whom we serve. We can, in fact, contribute to the fitness and health of older women in its broader definition while recognizing that they are our partners in this endeavor. After all, it is the old woman who has the greatest stake in the outcomes of our care and will generally help us if given the opportunity.

> I have a duty to all who care for me not to be a problem, not to be a burden. I must carry my age lightly for all our sakes, and thank God I still can.
>
> –F. Scott-Maxwell, 1968, p. 31

THE VERY OLD WOMAN

It is also important to mention very old women. Von Mehring (1992) writes about the rising "fourth age of life"–the population of great-grandparental age. These are the old-old and some of them reside in nursing homes; however, the vast majority of this group do not live in institutions and adapt well to their limitations (Wagnild & Young, 1990). They also find ways to live better with amazing fortitude and resourcefulness (von Mehring, 1992) and "they enlarge the possibilities and improve conditions for all women" (Thone, 1992). The importance of role modeling needs to be underscored. It is the women who are "enlarging the possibilities" in spite of handicaps and hardships that deserve our attention. However, research is now only beginning to appear about old-old women, the women of the "fourth age of life."

The future of older women seems to be viewed with optimism by some writers. Verbrugge (1985) writes, ". . . comparing a woman currently 75 years old with a woman that age in 2010, the future woman will probably feel better each day, have fewer disabilities, live longer and die more rapidly . . . Thus, we end with a positive view of future health for older women. The chances are that an older woman will have a more comfortable and active life than her same age peer today. And a larger fraction of U.S. females will reach older ages and have the opportunity to enjoy healthful old age" (pp. 63-64).

Although Birren (1978) was not writing about older women specifically, these prophetic words do apply well to this discussion. "Increasingly, in America, there will emerge a positive model of growing old. It will probably begin with the increasing awareness of older persons who 'have it together,' those who might be called the elite or accomplished aged. These are the people whom life refines and polishes. They move toward greater mastery of events and their adaptive strategies are such that they are increasingly strong and confident with the passage of years" (p. 206).

CONCLUSION

Health in older women has been considered from four perspectives of fitness: (a) physical, (b) intellectual, (c) social and (d) purpose fitness. While an older woman may not be fit in all of the four areas, certainly there are those who have become the elite and the polished old ones whom Birren described. It is not health, per se, which is so important in women's later lives, but the attitude, the stance they take toward their own health problems and their ability to cope, their finesse in meeting and adapting to new situations and crises which produces healthy older women. In spite of it all, they enlarge the possibilities for all women of all ages. The poet, Simon (1982), says it so well:

Craftswoman
See, she threads with bleeding feelings
The jagged shards of her shattered past.
From that which was tragedy
Or, at best, a grim joke.
Will she, can she weave
A design of grace?

REFERENCES

Birren, J.E. (1978). A gerontologist's overview. In L.F. Jarvik (Ed.). *Aging into the 21st Century.* New York: Gardner Press.

Birren, J.E., & Deutchman, D.E. (1991). *Guiding autobiography groups for older adults: Exploring the fabric of life.* Baltimore: The Johns Hopkins University Press.

Birren, J.E., & Zarit, J.M. (1985). Concepts of health, behavior and aging. In J.E. Birren & J. Livingston (Eds.). *Cognition, stress and aging* (pp. 1-20) Englewood Cliffs: Prentice-Hall.

Bould, S., Sanborn, B., & Reif, L. (1989). *Eighty-five plus: the oldest old.* Belmont, CA: Wadsworth Publishing.

Burnside, I. (1989). Groupwork with older women: a modality to improve the quality of life. In J.D. Garner & S.O. Mercer (Eds.). *Women as they age: Challenge, opportunity and triumph.* New York: The Haworth Press, Inc. pp. 265-280.

Burnside, I. (1990). *The effects of reminiscence groups on fatigue, affect and life satisfaction in older women.* Unpublished doctoral dissertation. The University of Texas, School of Nursing, Austin.

Burnside, I., & Schmidt, M.G. (In press). *Working with the elderly: Group process & technique* (3rd. ed.). Boston: Jones & Bartlett.

Butler, R. (1991). Forward in J.E. Birren & D.E. Deutchman (Eds.). *Guided autobiography groups: Exploring the fabric of life.* Baltimore: The Johns Hopkins University Press.

Carlson, A.D. (1977). *In the fullness of time: The pleasures and inconvenience of growing old.* Chicago: Henry Regnery Company.

de Beauvoir, S. (1972). *The coming of age.* New York: G.P. Putnam's Sons.

Garner, J.D. (1992). Personal letter.

Gordon, M. (1989). *Old enough to feel better.* Baltimore: Johns Hopkins University Press.

Hamilton, D.B. (1992). Reminiscence therapy in *Nursing interventions* (2nd ed). G.M. Bulechek, & J.C. McCloskey, (Eds.). Philadelphia: W.B. Saunders Company, pp. 292-303.

Knopf, O. (1975). *Successful aging: The facts and fallacies of growing old.* New York: Viking Press, Inc.

McCarthy, M.J. (1992). Home of one's own. *Wall Street Journal,* Vol. CXXVII, No. III, December 4, p.1.

Matteson, M.A., & McConnell, E.S. (1988). *Gerontological nursing: Concepts and practice*. Philadelphia: W. B. Saunders Company.

Mercer, S.O. & Garner, J.D. (1989). An international overview of aged women. In J.D. Garner & S.O., Mercer (Eds.). *Women as they age: Challenge, Opportunity and triumph*. New York: The Haworth Press, Inc., pp. 13-45.

Miller, C.A. (1990). *Nursing care of older adults: Theory and practice*. Glenview: Scott, Foresman/Little, Brown Higher Education.

Ouslander, J.G., & Beck, J.C. (1982). Defining the health problems of the elderly. *Annual Review of Public Health*, 3, 55-83.

Rhys, J. (1975). Whatever became of old Mrs. Pearce? *The Times*. London.

Rossman, I. (1988). *Looking Forward*. New York: E.P. Dutton.

Sands, J.O. (1981-82). The relationship of stressful life events to intellectual functioning in women over 65. *International Journal of Aging and Human Development 14*, 11-22.

Sarton, M. (1973). *Journal of solitude*, New York: W.W. Norton.

Sarton, M. (1980). *Recovering: A journal*, New York: W.W. Norton.

Sarton, M. (1984). *At seventy: A journal*, New York: W.W. Norton.

Schroot, J.J.F. (1988). Current perspectives on aging, health and behavior. In J.J.F. Schroot, J.E. Birren & A. Svanborg (Eds.). *Health and aging*. New York: Springer Publishing Company.

Scott-Maxwell, F. (1960). *The measure of my days*. New York: Alfred A. Knopf.

Simon, G. (1982). *In Late Harvest: Poems from Lifetime Learning of Newton*, The Coalition for Newton, Newton Community School, 492 Wartham Street, West Newton, MA.

Thone, R.R. (1992). *Women and aging: Celebrating ourselves*. New York: The Haworth Press, Inc.

U. S. Public Health Service (1991/1992). *Prevention report*. Dec/Jan: 1-2, 11.

Verbrugge, L.M. (1985). An epidemiological profile of older women. In M.R. Haug, A. B. Ford, M. Sheafor (Eds.). *The physical and mental health of aged women*. New York: The Springer Publishing Company.

Vinning, E. (1978). *Being seventy: The measure of a year*. New York: Viking Press.

Vischer, A.L. (1967). *On growing old*. Tr. by G. Onn. Boston: Houghton Mifflin Company.

Von Mering, O. (1992). Beyond the concept of successful aging: A transcultural and individual perspective. Conference, Successful aging–going beyond illness. Southern Regional Educational Board, Atlanta, GA.

Wagnild, G., & Young, H. (1990). Resilience among older women. *Image*, 22(4):252-255.

Webster's ninth new collegiate dictionary (1988). Springfield: Merriam-Webster, Inc.

After Menopause

Ann R. Peden, DSN, RN
Ann M. Newman, DSN, RN

SUMMARY. Women of 50 today have roughly the same number of years to look forward to as they have already lived as reproductive women. Many women will live 30, 40 or even 50 years post menopause. This very important period in women's lives has been studied little and viewed negatively by the medical profession and society at large. The purpose of this paper is to examine the psychological and physiological concerns of women at menopause. Self-help measures that are effective in managing the physical and psychological aspects of menopause are discussed. Hormone replacement therapy as a method of managing menopause is examined. Women are challenged to sort out the myths surrounding menopause, to take charge of their health and to move into this second season of their lives filled with vitality and joy.

Menopause is considered a life marker, the only universal symbol of transition, other than puberty, that is experienced by all women who live long enough. Menopause is no longer a marker that means "the way to the end." Today, menopause is viewed as the gateway to "Second Adulthood," and 50 is considered the peak

---

Ann R. Peden is Assistant Professor, College of Nursing, University of Kentucky, Lexington, KY.

Ann M. Newman is Assistant Professor of Nursing and Adjunct Professor of Women's Studies, College of Nursing, University of North Carolina, Charlotte, NC 28223.

[Haworth co-indexing entry note]: "After Menopause." Peden, Ann R., and Ann M. Newman. Co-published simultaneously in the *Journal of Women & Aging* (The Haworth Press, Inc.) Vol. 5, No. 3/4, 1993, pp. 25-40; and: *Women and Healthy Aging: Living Productively in Spite of It All.* (ed: J. Dianne Garner, and Alice A. Young), The Haworth Press, Inc., 1993, pp. 25-40. Multiple copies of this article/chapter may be purchased from The Haworth Document Delivery Center [1-800-3-HAWORTH; 9:00 a.m.-5:00 p.m. (EST)].

of the female life cycle. Women of 50 today have roughly the same number of years to look forward to as they have already lived as reproductive women. In fact, many women will live 30, 40 or even 50 years post menopause (Sheehy, 1992).

Yet, as frequently observed in the past decade, menopause is the period of women's lives least studied and least described in art, music, and literature. While it is often talked about, most often in a derogatory fashion, there is little indication that women are being listened to as they discuss menopause. A recent workshop hosted by a major university medical center featured a male physician expounding on menopause. Foremost on the program was a male physician who in a paper described, "The transition: What to expect." Where are the voices of women themselves?

According to Rosetta Reitz (1991), "menopause has had poor press. The bad parts have been touted and the good parts have been kept secret. Hot flashes and mood swings are TV fare for talk shows but they don't give equal time to the pleasure of no longer being burdened with a monthly flow of blood which must be absorbed or the freedom of sex without birth control" (p. xi). Roadmaps or standards against which to measure our own physiologic, psychologic and life changes are seriously lacking for women approaching menopause.

PSYCHOLOGICAL CONCERNS

Stereotypes

Because all women will experience menopause, and since it has increasingly come to be viewed as a "deficiency disease" (Greenblatt, 1974, p. 226) it is important to explore some of the largely unexamined assumptions which have the potential for impacting the lives of all women. With our cultural view of menopause and a health care system that focuses on illness care, it is no wonder that health care professionals have often viewed the natural event of menopause and menopausal women in a negative way. Medical myths do exist regarding menopause. Since women are major consumers of health care, this attitude has special implications for women. Fink (1988) suggested three things that influence the view of menopause as illness. These include the lack of quality medical research in the area of menopause, the large number of male physicians and the use of the diagnosis of menopause to cover a wide range of complaints of women between the ages of 40 and 65. In addition, it is not uncommon to find discussions of menopause in textbooks under the heading of diseases of estrogen deficiency (Harper, 1990).

Another common stereotype associated with menopausal women includes the view of menopause as an emotional crisis or period of instability. The myth was recently portrayed in the popular movie, "Fried Green Tomatoes" in which one of the characters, who was approaching menopause, exhibited periods of emotional instability and irrationality. The solution to her problem was summed up by "getting her some hormones." What the astute movie viewer actually saw was a woman who was making psychological changes which were going to occur with or without the aid of hormones.

Hot flashes, tears, accusations of women being victims of their hormones are all commonly used in routines delivered by stand-up comics or make up the story line in many popular situation comedies. The media bombards us with images of thin women, encouraging us to diet; even though we know that estrogen is stored in fat and that heavier women are less likely to develop osteoporosis. While obesity is not being encouraged, a moderate weight gain is not necessarily an unhealthy occurrence for the woman approaching menopause. Older women featured in films and television shows are for the most part youthful and thin. *Lear's,* a magazine designed for older women, features beautiful women on the cover and emphasizes success in their articles. However, for some women approaching menopause, new successful careers or other major changes may not be possible (Ginghofer, 1991).

Women are especially vulnerable to societal views as they approach and experience menopause. The years during which most women go through menopause are the same years in which multiple situational changes may occur. Children leave home, parents age and may become frail, a marriage that has lasted only for the children may end, an adulterous husband may be faced and retirement issues loom ahead. Coping mechanisms may already be stretched leaving reduced capacity to cope with the negative societal views toward menopause. It should come as no surprise that anxiety and depression may both be experienced by women at this time.

PHYSICAL CONCERNS

As estrogen levels decline, physical changes occur in a woman's body. The degree of discomfort that these changes cause are related to several factors, including age, rapidity at which estrogen is decreasing, body fat which stores estrogen and the woman's own interpretation of the symptoms (DeScharbo and Brucker, 1991). Vasomotor changes, vaginal changes, skin and hair changes and skeletal system changes will be discussed. Hormone replacement therapy is commonly used to treat these changes, although a great deal of controversy surrounds its widespread use.

Vasomotor Changes

Vasomotor changes are probably the first discomfort noted by many women who are menopausal. Commonly referred to as "hot flashes," this discomfort is experienced by 68% to 92% of perimenopausal women (Harper, 1990). It is described as a "sudden feeling of warmth in the head, neck and chest" (Lichtman, 1991, p. 32). It is often followed by a flush with perspiration and sometimes palpitations. Though not a sign of pathology, it is a disturbing symptom both physically and mentally.

According to Thompson, Hart, and Durno (1973), in a study of 90 women with hot flashes, over 68% experienced them daily, with 21% reporting them every few hours. The mean duration of the hot flash was 3.3 minutes with some lasting up to 60 minutes. Hot flashes are often accompanied by night sweats which interfere with sleep. The resulting sleep loss may lead to irritability and depression. These symptoms can occur four to six years after menopause and may begin years before menopause (Lichtman, 1991). Hot flashes may be triggered by alcohol, spicy foods, hot weather, emotional distress or a warm room.

Vaginal Changes

While estrogen does decline during menopause, androgens, the male hormones that affect sexual desire, continue to be produced.

Most menopausal women still continue to have strong sexual desires. However, in some women physiological changes that result from the loss of estrogen may interfere with pleasurable sexual encounters (Brady, 1990). The most common physiological change that effects sexuality is vaginal dryness.

The lining of the vagina is sensitive to the decreasing estrogen levels during the menopausal period. With decreasing estrogen levels, the vaginal epithelium becomes thinner. Vaginal lubrication and blood flow decrease. These changes manifest themselves with such vaginal discomforts as dryness, irritation, pain during sexual intercourse, and increase in vaginal infections. Vaginal ph changes also cause an increased risk of infection (Scharbo-DeHaan and Brucker, 1991).

For women who have vaginal dryness, sex-related pain makes a once pleasurable event one to be avoided. These physiological changes may also affect the woman's partner who fears causing pain and discomfort when engaging in sexual relations. Men at this age also may report declining sexual desire as a result of disease, age or lack of interest. But there is evidence that continued sexual activity can help maintain a woman's vaginal health. The adage, "use it or lose it," has relevance here. Women must be encouraged to seek help early with sexual problems that result from declining estrogen levels. Health care providers can help prevent sexual problems by the early dissemination of information about vaginal dryness. For most women, simply applying a vaginal lubricant relieves the problem. Open discussion with health care providers, provision of information and support will assist in normalizing this natural change. Early intervention can help maintain a woman's sexuality as she deals with successfully negotiating the menopausal period.

Skin and Hair Changes

The skin changes noted in women as they age include pigmentation changes, with too much resulting in darkened areas–sometimes referred to as "age spots"–or too little pigmentation which results in whitened or bleached areas. Dryness of skin, decreased elasticity and bruising are often reported (Scharbo-DeHaan and Brucker, 1991). It is not possible to determine whether these skin changes are solely the result of aging or menopause; it is interesting to note that men have the same changes. According to Greenwood (1989), the preventable effects of smoking and sun exposure are more likely to result in wrinkles.

Dry mouth is another discomfort reported by some women after menopause. Increased dental cavities and difficulty retaining dentures has also been noted. The mucosa that lines the mouth is affected by the decrease in estrogen.

A disturbing consequence of decreasing levels of estrogen in some women is the tendency to have thicker, coarser hair grow on the lip, chin, chest, and abdomen. If a woman has hair loss, it is likely to increase. These changes may also cause body image concerns in affected women.

Skeletal System Changes

As estrogen decreases, bone changes occur. Demineralization occurs at a greater rate than remineralization, causing women to be more susceptible to fractures. This pathologic condition is called osteoporosis and is more prevalent among certain groups of women. The typical woman at risk for osteoporosis is Caucasian or Oriental, slender and postmenopausal. Eagen (1989) reported that 5% to 10% of women will develop spinal fractures in the 25 years following menopause. The risk increases if there is a history of calcium deficiency, protein excess, substance abuses of alcohol, tobacco, and coffee, family history or medical disease associated with bone loss (Johnson, 1988). This woman's health problem is given an in-depth examination in a later section.

CHANGING BODY IMAGE

Also accompanying the physical changes associated with aging, and in women at the time of menopause are body image concerns. Most women have an ideal self that they incorporated into their being. It encompasses who they are and what they believe. With the physical changes that occur with aging, this ideal self is challenged. Since our culture values youth, society's view of the ideal woman is challenged as women age. That young woman with the beautiful skin and hair is no longer there. Wrinkles and gray hair stare back from the mirror. A restructuring of the ideal self must occur which incorporates the new, older self. This restructuring occurs as the woman confronts societal views of beauty, youth and aging. The belief that beauty can only be equated with youth must be discarded and replaced with the belief that aging women are beautiful. This restructuring may be difficult as women attempt to accept a new "older" ideal self.

According to Gail Sheehy, in her recent national best seller, *The Silent Passage: Menopause,* women must make an alliance with their changing bodies and their vanity, realizing that they will never be that idealized young woman again. The woman's task is to create a new future self that can be filled with trust and enthusiasm. A woman's second adulthood that begins at 50 has the potential to be her best.

STRATEGIES

Health Care Provider

Sheehy (1992), challenges women to find health care providers who will become partners during and after menopause. She encourages women, when seeking out that provider, whether it be a physician or nurse practitioner, to ask how many women over the age of 45 they treat. The answer to this question will provide information about the health care provider's interest or experience with menopausal women. Also, ask the provider to describe menopause. Listen to see if menopause is reduced to a list of symptoms or is referred to as a natural, normal process experienced by all women. The health care provider's view of menopause will affect the treatment approaches used. The willingness of the provider to answer questions should also be noted. If pat answers are received or questions brushed off, perhaps this is not the best health care provider for the menopausal woman.

When discussing medical tests, the ones to ask for are estrogen levels, LH and FSH levels and osteoporosis screening. "Be an inquiring, even challenging partner, not a passive follower of doctor-as-God. Decisions on how to plan for the health and well-being of your next 30 years or more cannot be made in a 20-minute office visit. Expect a year of trial and error" (Sheehy, 1991, p. 133). While finding the match with a health care provider may be expensive initially, it is well worth the effort.

As women enter this phase of their lives, they must be recognized as proactive health care consumers able to make informed choices about individual needs while choosing from a variety of health care services and providers. Health care decisions made by women in their early 50s will influence the quality of their life for the next 30 years. For this reason, these decisions must be made cautiously and prudently.

Hormone Replacement Therapy

Perhaps no greater controversy surrounds menopause than the use of Hormone Replacement Therapy (HRT). Women who are looking for answers about the benefits and risks of this medical intervention quickly realize that there are no clear answers. True, the use of Hormone Replacement Therapy does reduce the physical symptoms associated with menopause. Women report a decrease in hot flashes, a decrease in vaginal dryness and an overall sense of physical well-being while using HRT. A decrease in the occurrence of osteoporosis has also been linked with the use of HRT. However, this seemingly effective treatment carries with it risks. Women who were prescribed estrogen without the accompanying hormone progestogen were reported to develop endometrial cancer. This concern has diminished considerably with the addition of progestogen. The occurrence of breast malignancies may increase for women who take hormones; however, the research is not definitive and further study is needed (Lichtman, 1991).

HRT is associated with a reduced risk of cardiovascular disease in women (Stampfer, 1985). This raises the question of what benefits outweigh the risks. Researchers note that a woman has a greater chance of dying from heart disease than breast cancer. Studies on the long term effects of HRT are lacking. According to Dr. Lewis Kuller "it's the largest uncontrolled clinical trial in the history of medicine" (cited in Sheehy, 1992, p. 23). As the baby boomers age, it is estimated that a half million women each year for the next decade will move into the midlife population. The menopause market is big business. Drug companies estimate that hormones will account for close to a billion dollar market in 1992 (Sheehy, 1992). Becoming an informed consumer is the challenge that faces the women of this era.

Before HRT is chosen, the well-informed consumer will consider the following questions:

Is there a history of osteoporosis in your family?
Is there a history of breast cancer in your immediate relatives (mother or sister)?
Is there a family history of cancer of the uterus? (Sheehy, 1992)

When weighing the risks and benefits of HRT, risks to be considered include possible increased risk of cancer of uterus, unknown associations with breast cancer, continued menstruation is possible, breast swelling or pain, premenstrual-like syndrome on progesterone and expense of doctor's visits and tests for screening. Women on HRT are encouraged to undergo endometrial biopsy several months after starting hormones (Sheehy, 1992), to have routine mammograms, pelvic exams, stool guaiac and cholesterol and triglyceride levels (Mezrow and Rebar, 1988). The expense of doctor's visit and screening cannot be dismissed. Many women lack adequate financial or health care resources to manage these health promoting activities.

The benefits of HRT may include prevention of osteoporosis, heart disease, elimination of hot flashes, decreases in insomnia and restoration of sexual comfort. The best qualified person to determine if HRT is the appropriate treatment is the woman herself. She knows her stressors, lifestyle demands and family history. Hopefully with the increase in emphasis on the informed health care consumer, women will make informed decisions.

Self-Help Measures

For many women, there are other alternatives for coping with the changes that accompany menopause. Many involve vitamins, diet, exercise and the incorporation of health promoting activities.

Hot flashes are the most commonly reported symptom of menopause (Harper, 1990). They may continue for as long as six years after the last period. There are many practical things that women can do to assist in coping with this annoying symptom. Keeping cool is important for the woman experiencing hot flashes. Wear layered clothing that is easily removed. Avoid large meals. Caffeine, alcohol and strong emotions all make us warm. Drink cool beverages, be in cool rooms and eat small meals. These strategies will assist women in coping with hot flashes (Greenwood, 1984).

The use of Vitamin E has also been reported as relieving hot flashes. Vitamin E reduces the amount of FSH and LH in the woman's body. It should be taken after meals to aid absorption. It occurs naturally in wheat germ, whole grains, vegetable oils, soybeans, peanuts and spinach. The recommended dose is 100 IU initially, increasing over weeks or month to two to 600 IU until the hot flashes are relieved (Adams, 1986).

The herb, ginseng, is reported to increase feelings of well-being. Ginseng contains small amounts of estrogen. It should be used with caution in women who are diabetic or who have cardiac problems. The dose varies with body weight and it should be taken on an empty stomach, before or between meals. It may be purchased in health food stores. Prolonged use of ginseng has been known to cause hypertension; use cautiously (Greenwood, 1984).

Vitamin B complex is also useful in controlling hot flashes. It acts to detoxify and eliminate FSH which increases as estrogen decreases causing a shortening of the menstrual cycle and LH which affects ovulation (Scharbo-DeHaan and Brucker, 1991). It occurs in wheat germ and whole grains. It is also found in yogurt, brewer's yeast and milk. One to two vitamin tablets each day is recommended. Vitamin C and zinc have also been reported to aid in reducing hot flashes. The use of guided imagery and relaxation methods may also assist women in coping with this symptom.

Vaginal dryness and the accompanying changes affect a woman's sexual life. For many women, this period is one of sexual freedom. No longer is reproduction a concern, birth control a necessity. This freedom from the fear of conception gives many women a new perspective on their own sexuality. Women who have trouble with vaginal dryness and discomfort during intercourse can explain to

their partner the importance of adequate foreplay before intercourse. The use of water soluble jelly, coconut, vegetable or Vitamin E oil rubbed into the vagina daily and applied to the vagina and
penis prior to intercourse also reduces dryness (Greenwood, 1984).
A new product (Replens®) reportedly builds up a moist layer in the
vagina when used three times a week (Brody, 1990). Vaginal sup-
positories such as Lubrin® and Condom-mate® also provide mois-
ture when vaginal dryness is a problem. Many women report that
continued sexual activity, either masturbation or intercourse, reduce
vaginal soreness (Greenwood, 1984). Other measures include a hot
bath before intercourse, engaging in sexual activity in the morning
when more rested, the woman astride to control penetration and the
use of erotica, films or books (Bachman, 1988).

A daily supplement of Zinc (15 mg) and non-medical treatment of
vaginal infections may also decrease the incidence of vaginal infections. Non-medical treatments include cotton underwear, use of sitz
baths and yogurt douche (Scharbo-DeHaan and Brucker, 1991). Certain drugs can contribute to vaginal dryness and may inhibit sexuality
in other ways. These include antidepressants, diuretics, barbiturates,
antihistamines and phenothiazines (Steege, 1986).

Wrinkling of the skin is more than likely the result of sun exposure and smoking rather than aging and menopause. Treatments for
dry skin include lotion and oils that don't contain alcohol. Dry
mouth can be relieved by good dental hygiene, gum massage and
the use of breath mints (Scharbo-DeHaan and Brucker, 1991).
Unwanted hair may be removed by electrolysis, topical creams,
tweezing, shaving or simply bleaching the hair to make it less
noticeable. The method for removing unwanted hair should be left
up to the woman.

Diet and exercise are the most commonly recommended interventions to decrease skeletal system changes. According to Greenwood (1984), a diet high in vegetables, whole grains, fruit and
foods high in calcium will supply necessary nutrients and not cause
obesity or heart disease. Proper diet can result in an increase in
energy, weight stabilization, healthy hair, skin and gums.

Exercise in combination with adequate dietary calcium can build
bone and slow bone loss. Exercise that puts traction on long bones
is recommended. These include walking, tennis, dancing and bik-

ing. A diet rich in calcium includes milk, cheese, yogurt, green vegetables, sesame seeds, maple syrup and turnip greens. Calcium supplements are also available. To prevent bone loss, it is recommended that young women take 1 gram of calcium per day. Postmenopausal women increase their dosage to 1.5 grams per day (Adams, 1986).

Replacing the Stereotypes

Something as powerful and pervasive as ageism is internalized to one extent or another by all. It is no wonder that stereotypes abound and so influence us. The blatant stereotypes are the most amenable to change. The more subtle stereotypes are more eroding to self-esteem and more limiting to life experience. Despite the stereotypes, women after menopause often take greater risks, have less concern with approval, reevaluate the meaning of success, become increasingly independent and find new dimensions to their sexual being. These are the behaviors that must be modeled by older women thus replacing those old stereotypes.

It is not enough to reject the negative stereotypes held by our society. They must be replaced by positive strong images. It is the responsibility of older women to provide these–showing younger women how healthy and powerful the later years can become. A whole new life opens up as women use their experience and knowledge to improve our world (Mickelson, 1991).

Mastering the Psychosocial Challenges

Sheehy (1992) has coined the phrase, coalescence, to describe a woman's new state once the ovarian transition is complete. This state culminates in a coming together of energy, moods, and an overall sense of physical and mental well-being. As women move beyond the stereotypes of sexual object and breeder, they become free to speak their minds and initiate action. This move is cause for celebration.

Women at this period of life must find their passion, be it politics, returning to school, hobbies, relationships, writing or whatever provides challenge and pleasure. "It is essential to claim the pause and find this new source of aliveness and meaning that will make the years ahead even more precious than those past" (Sheehy, 1992, p. 140). Welcoming post-menopause, being energized by this change, preparing for the new freedoms that accompany it will affect a woman's psychological response to this time of life. A woman's body is no longer faced with monthly hormone surges. Progesterone no longer fluctuates and women no longer experience the mood swings associated with the menstrual years. Perhaps it is this physiological change that provides women with this new energy experienced in post menopause (Sheehy, 1992).

Psychological Self-Help Measures

To successfully master the psychological challenges associated with this life transition, women must learn how to tune down stress which can have negative effects on their hearts, keep the minerals in their bones and visualize their ideal self with wrinkles and graying hair (Sheehy, 1992). Adopting a healthy attitude about menopause will result in a healthier woman. As discussed earlier, this may be difficult due to the societal view of menopausal women as being past their prime. But with the graying of America, comes large numbers of women who are very much in their prime. The sheer numbers of menopausal and post-menopausal women are forcing society to reevaluate its negative stereotypes of older women. Self-help groups are emerging that have the potential to help ourselves and others (Mickelson, 1991).

Participation in a menopause support group is one way in which women can garner the support and encouragement needed as they make this life transition. A support group can lend reassurance about normal physical changes, but also provide emotional encouragement as well as provide new direction in women's lives. This time in life allows women the time to reevaluate, to focus on self rather than family or career. Opportunity is provided for a woman to go into herself and realize what her values are and what she hopes to get out of the rest of her life. The focus is on building up, adding to what the person already is. For many women, this focus becomes one of service to others.

But service to others is not limited to altruistic pursuits, it may be interpreted as a return to school, a new job or picking up a career that has been on hold. There is more time to share with spouse, perhaps renewing that one-to-one relationship which existed before children (Mickelson, 1991). "Menopause offers us an opportunity to appreciate and nurture ourselves, to devote time to seeking the right physical and emotional balance for us. It's a time to reawaken old friendships and to foster new friendships, which will enrich our lives for years to come. Menopause provides the impetus to get to know ourselves more intimately, a self-knowledge that is invaluable as we face the challenge of aging" (Cobb, 1991, p. 29).

Research on Menopause

Little research has been done on healthy menopausal women. Opportunities for research include epidemiological studies of healthy women experiencing normal aging, studies to determine if surgical menopause contributes to poor health and studies of the effects of the health care professional's stereotypes on the delivery of care to menopausal women. Qualitative studies that examine the experiences of culture and ethnicity in mid-life women are needed. Also lacking in current research literature are longitudinal cohort studies of post-menopausal women who do or do not take Hormone Replacement Therapy and studies of the cumulative effects of years of birth control and hormone replacement therapy. Finally, qualitative studies that reflect women's experiences surrounding menopause with an emphasis on the post-menopausal woman are needed. There is much to be learned from post-menopausal women about their entry into this second adulthood. By careful listening, road maps or guidance may be provided that can guide all women as they move through this life change.

CONCLUSION

The changes associated with menopause are largely controllable. Good nutrition, exercise and the avoidance of undue stress can affect menopause. Women must be encouraged to treat themselves with the same care and wonder with which they treated their pregnant or nursing body. Involving self with people, forming strong support systems and providing positive role models for younger women will also make the transition into the second adulthood easier.

There are 43 million American women either undergoing or past menopause (Sheehy, 1992). With the "graying" of the American population, and the fact that women usually outlive men, women must learn to be vigilant in sorting out the myths surrounding menopause, taking charge of their health, and moving towards the ultimate goal of living a richer and fuller life. Menopause is not a deficiency disease–it should be experienced with joie de vivre as the gateway to a "Second Adulthood."

REFERENCES

Adams, B.N. (1986). The middle years woman: Education for health promotion and maintenance. In V. M. Littlefield (Ed.), *Health education for women: A guide for nurses and other health professionals* (pp. 336-337). Norwalk, CT: Appleton-Century-Crofts.

Bachmann, G.A. (1988). Sexual dysfunction in postmenopausal women: The role of medical management. *Geriatrics, 43,* 79-83.

Brody, J.E. (1990, May 10). Personal health: On menopause and the toll that loss of estrogens can take on a woman's sexuality. *The New York Times,* p. B15.

Cobb, J.O. (1991). The impetus of menopause. In D. Taylor & A.C. Sumrall (Eds.), *Women of the 14th moon* (pp. 26-29). Freedom, CA: Crossing Press.

Eagen, A. (1989, May-June). Reconsidering hormone replacement therapy. *The Network News,* 3-5.

Fink, P.J. (1988). Psychiatric myths of menopause. In B.A. Eskin (Ed.), *Menopause: Comprehensive management* (2nd ed.). New York: Macmillan.

Ginghofer, J.J. (1991). Sex, signs, and media-hype. In D. Taylor & A.C. Sumrall (Eds.), *Women of the 14th moon* (pp. 226-231). Freedom, CA: Crossing Press.

Greenblatt, R. (1974). Reprise. In R. Greenblatt, V. Mahesh, & P. McDonough (Eds.), *Menopausal syndrome* (pp. 223-231). New York: Medcom Press.

Greenwood, S. (1984). *Menopause naturally.* San Francisco: Volcano Press.

Harper, D. (1990). Perimenopause and aging. In R. Lichtman & S. Papera (Eds.), *Gynecology: Well-woman care.* Chicago: Year Book Medical.

Johnson, C.C. (1988). Osteoporosis. In B.A. Eskin (Ed.), *Menopause: Comprehensive management* (2nd ed.). New York: Macmillan.

Lichtman, R. (1991). Perimenopausal hormone replacement therapy. *Journal of Nurse-Midwifery, 36,* 30-44.

Mezrow, G. & Rebar, R.W. (1988). Tailoring estrogen replacement to fit the patient. *Contemporary Obstetrics/Gynecology, 31,* 51-60.

Mickelson, J.L. (1991). Changing woman. In D. Taylor & A.C. Sumrall (Eds.), *Women of the 14th moon* (pp. 33-39). Freedom, CA: Crossing Press.

Reitz, R. (1991). Foreward. In D. Taylor & A.C. Sumrall (Eds.), *Women of the 14th moon* (pp. xi-xiv). Freedom, CA: Crossing Press.

Scharbo-DeHaan, M.S. & Brucker, M.C. (1991). The perimenopausal period: Implications for nurse-midwifery practice. *Journal of Nurse-Midwifery, 36,* 9-16.

Sheehy, G. (1992). *The silent passage: Menopause.* New York: Random House.

Stampfer, M. (1985). A prospective study of postmenopausal estrogen therapy and coronary heart disease. *New England Journal of Medicine, 313,* 1044-1049.

Steege, J.F. (1986). Sexual function in the aging woman. *Clinical Obstetrics & Gynecology, 29,* 462-469.

Thompson, B., Hart, S.A., & Durno, D. (1973). Menopausal age and symptomatology in a general practice. *Journal of Biosocial Science, 5,* 71-82.

Menopause

Thirty experiences year after year
sisterhood of blood accustomed rhythms
reassuring flow disappointing flow.
I will not be like those old women
I try not to see.

Fifty inquires when the blood ceases
what else will leave when the blood dries
what else will dry when the hot flashes
burn away desire.
Will he leave me will I lose me
what will old age be?

Seventy responds we are not bloodless
we have new rhythms our life force flows
love does not cease desire does not dry
hot flashes of wit prove we are not lost
we birth crone's wisdom
see us hear our glee.

–Ruth Harriet Jacobs, PhD

Ruth Harriet Jacobs is Researcher, Wellesley College Center for Research on Women, Wellesley, MA 02181.

[Haworth co-indexing entry note]: "Menopause." Jacobs, Ruth Harriet. Co-published simultaneously in the *Journal of Women & Aging* (The Haworth Press, Inc.) Vol. 5, No. 3/4, 1993, p. 41; and: *Women and Healthy Aging: Living Productively in Spite of It All* (ed: J. Dianne Garner, and Alice A. Young), The Haworth Press, Inc., 1993, p. 41. Multiple copies of this article/chapter may be purchased from The Haworth Document Delivery Center [1-800-3-HAWORTH; 9:00 a.m.-5:00 p.m. (EST)].

Osteoporosis and Older Women: Productive Lifestyle Strategies

Karen A. Roberto, PhD

SUMMARY. Osteoporosis, a metabolic bone disorder, affects four times as many women as men. Each year 1.3 million fractures, primarily of the vertebra, hip, and wrist can be attributed to osteoporosis. Risk factors for the development of this disease include age, sex, body build, family history, race, loss of estrogen, calcium deficiency, sedentary lifestyle, smoking, and the excessive use of alcohol. Three common approaches used in the treatment and prevention of osteoporosis are hormone replacement therapies, nutrition interventions, and exercise programs. These strategies are aimed at maintaining or stabilizing bone mass and preventing further loss. Living with osteoporosis presents older women with a variety of physical, psychological, and social challenges. To maintain a productive and healthy lifestyle, older women must recognize their physical limitations and make adjustments in their daily lives to cope successfully with these changes.

Osteoporosis is a metabolic bone disorder characterized by a gradual reduction in bone mass to the point that microscopic or more obvious fracturing occurs. This condition affects over 25 million Americans, including four times as many women as men (National Osteoporosis Foundation [NOF], 1991). Each year 1.3 million frac-

Karen A. Roberto is Associate Professor and Coordinator, Gerontology Program, University of Northern Colorado, Greeley, CO 80639.

[Haworth co-indexing entry note]: "Osteoporosis and Older Women: Productive Lifestyle Strategies." Roberto, Karen A. Co-published simultaneously in the *Journal of Women & Aging* (The Haworth Press, Inc.) Vol. 5, No. 3/4, 1993, pp. 43-59; and: *Women and Healthy Aging: Living Productively in Spite of It All* (ed: J. Dianne Garner, and Alice A. Young), The Haworth Press, Inc., 1993, pp. 43-59. Multiple copies of this article/chapter may be purchased from The Haworth Document Delivery Center [1-800-3-HAWORTH; 9:00 a.m.-5:00 p.m. (EST)].

43

tures, primarily of the vertebra (500,000), hip (250,000), and wrist (170,000) may be attributed to osteoporosis (Department of Health and Human Services [DHHS], 1991). Although hip fractures cause the greatest disability, fractures of the vertebra, humerus, and pelvis also cause considerable morbidity.

The estimated annual cost of osteoporosis in the United States is between 7 to 10 billion dollars. This enormous economic burden stems from the millions of restricted activity days, the millions of days in hospitals, and nearly a million physician office visits experienced by individuals with osteoporosis (DHHS, 1991). What the financial figures do not take into account, however, is the physical (e.g., pain), psychological (e.g., poor self-concept; low self-esteem) and social (e.g., dependency on others, limited socialization) costs of living with this devastating disease.

The all-encompassing nature of osteoporosis requires an understanding of information from both the biomedical and psychosocial research arenas. Specific topics to be addressed include: (1) risk factors for developing osteoporosis, (2) the disease process, (3) prevention and treatment options, and (4) strategies for coping with osteoporosis to promote a productive and healthy aging.

RISK FACTORS FOR OSTEOPOROSIS

Risk for osteoporosis depends mainly upon peak adult bone density and its subsequent rate of loss (Whitcroft & Stevenson, 1992). A variety of non-modifiable and modifiable factors influence the formation and maintenance of sufficient bone mass and place individuals at risk for the development of osteoporosis.

Non-Modifiable Risks

Age, sex, body build, family history, and race are the commonly cited non-modifiable risk factors for the development of osteoporosis (Albers, 1990; Heidrich & Thompson, 1987; Miller, 1992; NOF, 1991). During the third decade, all individuals begin to experience a gradual lose of bone mass (Bourguet, Hamrick, & Gilchrist, 1991; Sagraves, 1991). This decline results in weaker bone structure and creates greater susceptibility to osteoporotic fractures. Since women tend to start out with a lower peak bone mass than men and have accelerated bone mass loss following menopause, they are four times as likely to develop osteoporosis than their male counterparts. Short, small-boned women have a greater likelihood of developing osteoporosis because they have less total bone mass at maturity. Low bone mass may be a result of heredity. One group of scientists reported that daughters of women with postmenopausal osteoporosis had lower spinal bone mass than daughters of women who were not osteoporotic (Seeman, Hopper, Bach, Cooper, Parkinson, McKay, & Jerums, 1989). Caucasians and Asian individuals also have a higher incidence of osteoporosis than darker-skinned persons.

Modifiable Risks

Several modifiable risk factors also are associated with the development of osteoporosis. These include: loss of estrogen, calcium deficiency, sedentary lifestyle, smoking, excessive use of alcohol and caffeine, and the use of certain medications (Miller, 1992; Smith, 1992). For example, the loss of estrogen when menstruation ceases results in accelerated bone loss. Individuals with osteoporosis tend to have lower levels of calcium intake than persons without the disease (Santora, 1987). Lack of weight-bearing exercise, smoking, and the excessive use of alcohol and caffeine contribute to a loss of bone mass and an increased risk of osteoporotic fractures. In addition, excessive or long-term use of certain medications, such as steroids and diuretics, interferes with the absorption of nutrients and may contribute to the reduction of overall bone mass (Heidrich & Thompson, 1987; Miller, 1992).

THE DISEASE PROCESS

Bone Remodeling

Bone remodeling, or the formation and resorption of bone, continually occurs throughout a person's lifetime. Simply put, the sequence of remodeling begins with the activation of osteoclasts. Osteoclasts dig microscopic cavities in the inner surface of the bone and resorb a small amount of the bone. Next, osteoblasts appear and deposit new bone cells in the cavities. After the osteoblasts are in place, the mineralization of bone begins. The entire remodeling process takes approximately four months with an estimated 10 to 30 percent of a person's bone replaced annually (Notelovitz & Ware, 1985).

Although the rate of remodeling differs for various portions of the skeleton, the formation and resorption of bone is a balanced, or tightly coupled process through the third decade of life (DHHS, 1991). In the fourth decade, however, bone mass begins to decline because bone formation cannot keep up with bone resorption. For a variety of reasons, including lower peak bone mass and estrogen withdrawal at menopause, women are more susceptible to the consequences of abnormal remodeling.

Types of Bone Loss and Osteoporosis

The human skeleton is comprised of approximately 20% trabecular bone, the honeycombed, interior meshwork of the bone, and 80% cortical bone, the dense, outer shell of the skeleton. Women lose trabecular bone mass more rapidly than men. By the time a woman reaches 80, she will have lost approximately 47% of her trabecular bone while her male counterpart will have lost only about 14% of his trabecular bone mass (Notelovitz & Ware, 1985). Both men and women experience a slight loss of cortical bone throughout their life-time. During menopause, however, women lose cortical bone mass at a much accelerated rate. In general, menopause accounts for a 10 to 15% reduction of cortical bone mass loss (Genant, Baylink, & Gallagher, 1989).

The difference in bone mass loss has led some researchers to distinguish between two types of osteoporosis (Riggs & Melton, 1986; Smith, 1992). Type I, or postmenopausal osteoporosis, results primarily from the loss of trabecular bone in the vertebra and distal forearm. As a result of the loss of estrogen, women between the ages 51 to 70 are six times more suspectable to this type of osteoporosis than men. Type II, or senile osteoporosis, occurs in individuals over age 70 and is attributed to the process of aging. About twice as many women than men suffer hip, vertebral, humerus, and pelvic fractures because of the slow loss of both trabecular and cortical bone that is characteristic of senile osteoporosis.

Detection

Osteoporosis is called the "silent disease" since diagnosis often comes only after an older person sustains a fracture. X-rays are useful to detect breaks in bones, but they are not sensitive enough to detect osteoporosis until at least 25 to 30 percent of bone mass is depleted (Miller, 1992). By this time, the disease is in an advanced stage.

Innovative medical technology, however, provides physicians with more sensitive, diagnostic tests by which to measure bone mass in various sites in the body and to predict the likelihood of future fractures. Tests vary with respect to the site measured, precision, accuracy, time required, dose of radiation, and cost (DHHS, 1991; NOF, 1991; Smith, 1992). For example, the *single energy photon absorptiometry* (SPA) is primarily used to measure cortical bone sites such as the wrist, forearm, and heel. It is a relatively fast, inexpensive, and sensitive technique. The *dual photon absorptiometry* (DPA) takes measures of the spine, hip, and whole body. Although standard screening is slow, this technique has good accuracy and precision. The vertebra is the site of measurement for the *quantitative computed tomography* (QCT). Although it is fairly precise, this technique uses a higher radiation dose than most other instruments. The *dual x-ray absorptiometry* (DXA) measures bone tissue in the hip and spine. This instrument represents a major diagnostic advancement for following patients and for monitoring therapy as it is precise enough to detect a one to two percent loss or gain of bone mass (Miller, 1992).

Progression

McIlwain and his colleagues (1988) describe four stages in the progression of osteoporosis. The first stage begins between the age of 30 and 40 with a gradual decrease in the total amount of bone mass in the body. The loss is slow and is not possible to detect.

Stage 2 usually begins sometime after age 35 and continues through age 55. There has been a gradual loss of bone for several years, but the remaining bone is still strong. Fractures during this period are unusual. Although there are no noticeable signs or symptoms of osteoporosis, it is in this stage that it first becomes detectable through advanced testing techniques (e.g., absorptiometry and tomography).

Stage 3 usually begins sometime after age 55. A fractured bone marks its onset. The fracture may result from a minor fall or strain. Pain, attributed to osteoporosis, often occurs during this stage. Although acute pain is common with all types of fracture, the pain associated with the occurrence of vertebral fractures may be of a longer duration.

If the disease progresses to stage 4, a person's bones become increasingly brittle. This results in an increase in the number of fractures, pain, loss of height, and the development of visible physical deformities such as a protruding stomach or dowager's hump.

MEDICAL PREVENTION AND TREATMENT OPTIONS

Currently, there is not a cure for osteoporosis. Available treatment modalities are aimed at maintaining or stabilizing bone mass and preventing further loss. With the use of advanced screening measures, it is possible to detect osteoporosis in its early stages, before any symptoms of pain or fractures occur. Two common approaches used in the treatment and prevention of osteoporosis are hormone replacement therapies and nutrition interventions.

Hormone Therapies

Estrogen Replacement Therapy (ERT). Menopause-related estrogen deficiency is responsible for one-third to one-half of the bone loss during a woman's lifetime (Genant et al., 1989). The administration of estrogen reduces the rate of bone resorption and facilitates normal bone remodeling. Positive effects on bone, such as equilibration of bone resorption and formation and the stabilization of bone mass, are noted within 6 to 24 months of beginning ERT (Sagraves, 1991). Although many studies support the efficiency of ERT in reducing fractures, it does not restore lost bone mass. Women with poor skeletal density at menopause, therefore, may still be at risk for fractures even with ERT (Genant et al., 1989). In addition, estrogen delays bone mass loss only for as long as it is used. Stopping therapy results in resumption of bone loss and increases the risk of fracture (Heidrich & Thompson, 1987; Quigley, Martin, Burnier, & Brooks, 1987).

Experts differ in their opinions on when women should begin ERT and on the duration of treatment. Stevenson and his colleagues (1989) suggest that ERT started early in the menopause process and continued for at least five years decreases the general incidence of osteoporotic fractures by at least fifty percent. Others suggest that ERT may still be effective even if started up to 15 years after menopause with women who have high bone mass loss and Type I osteoporosis (Riggs & Melton, 1986). No conclusive guidelines exist as to the length of time ERT should be administered. Some physicians consider ERT a lifelong therapy for women, while others do not recommend ERT for women over the age of 75 (McKeon, 1990).

ERT usually is administered orally. The high concentration of estrogen in the woman's system after oral administration reportedly accounts for several complications associated with ERT. An alternative approach, transdermal administration, provides a continuous release of estrogen into the circulatory system. This may prevent some of the complications associated with ERT (McKeon, 1990). ERT, via transdermal administration, is as effective as orally administered estrogen in preventing bone loss. Researchers report that transdermal ERT given to peri-menopausal women prevents postmenopausal bone loss (Stevenson, Anst, Gangar, Hillard, Lees, & Whitehead, 1990) and stabilizes bone loss in postmenopausal women with established osteoporosis (Lufkin et al., 1992).

Despite the clear benefits of ERT, less than 18% of the 40 million women who are eligible for ERT actually take it (Munnings, 1992). The potential risks associated with the hormonal regime may deter some women and their physicians from beginning ERT. These risks included increases in the development of (1) endometrial, breast, and ovarian cancer; (2) hypertension; (3) gall-bladder disease; and (4) glucose intolerance (McKeon, 1990; Sagraves, 1991; Whitcroft & Stevenson, 1992). Controversy exists, however, as to whether these are true risks, particularly around the increase of breast cancer. Two recent meta-analyses of studies reporting an association between the use of ERT and breast cancer counters the original findings (Dupont & Page, 1991; Steinberg et al., 1991).

Other adverse effects, although not life-threatening, include bloating, breast tenderness, abdominal cramps, and withdrawal bleeding (McKeon, 1992). The use of progesterone in conjunction with ERT may cause premenstrual tension-like symptoms such as irritability, anxiety, and depression. These adverse effects often result in noncompliance with the therapeutic regime.

Calcitonin. Calcitonin, a hormone that slows bone breakdown, has been used for treating established osteoporosis in both men and women. Calcitonin increases skeletal density about 6 to 10% within the first year of use but produces no further increases thereafter (Licata, 1991). It also has an analgesic property that is effective in relieving severe skeletal pain.

Nutrition Interventions

Calcium. The recommended daily allowance (RDA) for calcium for non-pregnant, nonlactating adults is 800 mg per day. Calcium intakes, particularly for women, are typically lower. After age 35, 75% of all females have calcium intakes below the RDA (Ramazzotto, Curro, Gates, & Patterson, 1986). In addition, there is some indication that calcium requirements increase with age. Based on these estimates, the 1984 Consensus Conference on Osteoporosis approved an increase in the RDA of 1000 mg/day for estrogen replete and 1500 mg per day for estrogen deprived women.

The potential effectiveness of high intakes of calcium for the prevention and treatment of osteoporosis is a matter of debate among professionals. Based on a review of clinical and intervention studies, Bales (1990) concluded that a clear relationship between low calcium intake and bone loss does not exist. She noted that although several investigators indicated that women with osteoporosis report lower calcium intakes than controls, others have not found this relationship. The research suggests similar contradictions for calcium supplements. Some researchers report positive effects of over-the-counter calcium supplementation on the bone density of older women, while others report little or no effects. Differences in findings may be a result of comparing bone loss from different skeletal sites, the wide range of calcium intakes, and the point during the menopausal period in which calcium treatment begins (Bales, 1990; Sagraves, 1991).

Although there are a variety of calcium products available, some researchers suggest that calcium carbonate has several advantages over other supplements. This supplement contains the largest percentage of calcium, has a good absorption rate, and typically is less expensive to use than other calcium supplements (Gossel, 1991). The formation of kidney stones is one risk of using calcium supplements, particularly for persons with hypercalcemia. Adverse effects, such as nausea, constipation, excess gas and bloating, are rare (Gossel, 1991).

Vitamin D. Vitamin D plays a central role in calcium absorption and incorporation into the bone. Typically, it is given to persons who have an inability to absorb calcium properly. There is evidence that modest increases in bone density and thus the prevention of osteoporosis occurs with the use of vitamin D analogs (DHHS, 1991). The DHHS report also suggests that vitamin D analogs are effective in reducing vertebral fracture rate. High doses of vitamin D, however, cause negative side effects such as hypercalcemia, hypercalciuria, and kidney stones (Fujita, 1992).

Fluoride. Most of the current treatments for osteoporosis work to slow bone resorption but have little effect on stimulating bone formation. Sodium fluoride is the exception. Clinical studies suggest that fluoride has the potential to produce sustained improvement in trabecular bone volume (Eriksen, Hodgson, & Riggs, 1988). There appears, however, to be considerable variation in response to fluoride treatments, with 30% of individuals treated showing little or no positive gains in bone apposition (DHHS, 1991). Many women, however, cannot tolerate fluoride supplements. Adverse effects include nausea, gastric irritation, lower extremity pain. Perhaps more worrisome is the suggestion that bone formed during the administration of fluoride may be less strong and more fragile than normal bone (Riggs et al., 1990).

Bisphosphonates. Bisphosphonates appear to decrease bone resorption without a corresponding decrease in formation. This results in a net accrual of bone mass and thereby a reduction in new fracture rate (DHHS, 1991). Etidronate disodium is one of five bisphosphonates under investigation for the treatment of osteoporosis. Short-term studies of one-to-three years indicate its effectiveness in increasing bone density and reducing fractures by over 50 percent (Licata, 1991). The long-term risks and benefits, the most effective therapeutic program (i.e., continuous or sequential), and appropriate dosage for the bisphosphonates have yet to be determined (DHHS, 1991).

STRATEGIES FOR A PRODUCTIVE
AND HEALTHY AGING

A diagnosis of osteoporosis presents older women with a variety of physical, psychological, and social challenges. To maintain a productive and healthy lifestyle, older women must recognize their physical limitations and make adjustments in their lives to manage these changes. The nature of the disease requires the use of both physical and psychosocial strategies to successfully cope with these lifestyle issues.

Physical Strategies

Exercise. Exercise plays an important role in stimulating the bone remodeling cycle. Researchers suggest that consistent participation in weight-bearing activities such as walking, jogging, weight-training, and aerobic exercise maximize and maintain bone mass in both pre- and postmenopausal women (Munnings, 1992; Shangold, 1990). The increased strength that women develop because of their involvement in exercise programs also may reduce the likelihood of falls. This is an important benefit since 90% of all osteoporotic fractures are fall related and as many as one-third of women between the ages of 65 and 74 fall each year (Munnings, 1992).

A combination of vigorous aerobic and strength training, started early in life, is an effective strategy for the prevention of osteoporosis (Gutin & Kasper, 1992). If maintained, this type of regime also helps reduce age-related bone loss in later years. Although there is no set prescription for the amount of exercise necessary to prevent or delay osteoporosis, if women decrease or stop their exercising, their rate of bone mass loss increases (Munnings, 1992).

The relationship between exercise and other treatment strategies is not clear. Some researchers indicate that exercise is more effective when used with ERT or calcium supplementation, while others report no interactive effects (Gutin & Kasper, 1992).

Diet. A healthy lifestyle requires a well-balanced diet. The development and maintenance of a sound bone structure requires an intake of a variety of nutrients, including calcium, vitamin D and fluoride. Dietary calcium is preferred to supplemental sources because of the additional vitamins, minerals, and trace elements acquired through food. Dairy products provide the best dietary sources of calcium, supplying 75% of calcium intakes in the United States (Bales, 1990).

Psychosocial Strategies

Personal Management. Living with osteoporosis requires older women to make adjustments in all aspects of their lives (Roberto, 1988; 1989; 1990). For example, the intense pain, associated with osteoporosis is often remedied by taking pain relievers, lying down and resting, and using a heating pad or taking a hot bath (Hallal, 1991; Roberto, 1989). To manage physical restrictions or impairments, women may need to use supportive devices (e.g., back brace, cane, and walker). Osteoporosis can also impact the sleep and rest patterns of older women. Scheduled rest periods throughout the day may be helpful as well as necessary, especially for women who have their night-time sleep patterns disrupted. Some women find switching from a firm mattress to a waterbed improves their ability to sleep.

Living with osteoporosis also may require a change in family responsibilities. As a result of decreased functional abilities, many women with osteoporosis need to modify their household duties, particularly those requiring reaching, lifting, pulling, or shoving in order not to aggravate their condition. Redefining their "housekeeper" role, however, is especially difficult for women who view the home as their domain (Roberto, 1988). For example, one woman with osteoporosis reported that although she was grateful that her husband was willing to do some of her chores, her "floors sure don't sparkle like they use to!" To guard against feelings of uselessness and dependency, older women must learn to recognize and work within their physical limits to achieve their maximum level of productivity. For many women this means pacing themselves and incorporating "break time" into their daily routines.

Women with osteoporosis often must alter their social and recreational activities. Depending on the situation, the amount of physical energy and mobility required, and their personalities, women use different ways of coping. Unfortunately, some women automatically give up activities that they once enjoyed. A more satisfying approach for many women is to make adjustments in the frequency or intensity of their social and recreational involvements (Roberto, 1990). For example, one woman described how, prior to the onset of her osteoporosis, she had a "shopping day" where she would go from store to store. Now, she often shops several times a week, but only goes to one store a day. The development of new skills or interests, that do not place unnecessary stress on the skeletal system, is another means by which women with osteoporosis can sustain their opportunities for recreational activities and social interactions (Roberto & Johnston, 1991).

The progressive nature of osteoporosis requires women continually to make short and long-term adjustments in their lifestyles. These changes can increase stress levels (Roberto, 1989), induce feelings of depression, and alter the woman's sense of self (Roberto & McGraw, 1991). These psychological manifestations should not be ignored as they can impede the woman's coping abilities. Older women are encouraged to use a variety of coping strategies including information seeking, direct action, inhibition of action, and intrapsychic responses (e.g., humor) to handle the stress of osteoporosis (Gold, Lyles, Bales, & Drezner, 1989).

Reliance on Family and Friends. Family members and friends play an important role in providing assistance and emotional support to older persons with chronic health conditions. Women with osteoporosis report depending on their spouses, children, and to some extent siblings to help them with tasks that have become too difficult to carry out (Roberto, 1988). Assistance with daily tasks is more frequent when a woman has sustained a fracture and the impact of her osteoporosis is more evident. The association of need for assistance with visible cues is unfortunate, particularly with a condition such as osteoporosis where pain may limit a woman's abilities even though an overt fracture has not occurred. Having a physician set specific limits on the women's daily activities may help them explain their condition to family members and facilitate the family's acceptance of the disease (Gold et al., 1989).

Osteoporosis also influences the quality of the women's relationship with their family and friends. Sustaining a fracture or continual pain may inhibit women from interacting with others or from participating in activities with their informal network. The more problems created by the disease, the less women perceive themselves as integrated within their social network (Roberto & Johnston, 1991). Feelings of belonging provided by a social support system are important in preventing psychological distress (e.g., loneliness, isolation, depression) often associated with long-term illness (Cohen & McKay, 1984). Women with osteoporosis, therefore, should be encouraged to maintain some level of involvement with members of their social network. The development of new relationships can also strengthen or sustain the women's feelings of self-worth. For example, joining an osteoporosis support group can provide women the opportunity to extend their social network as well as influence the well-being of another person. This type of interaction can be very satisfying and add meaning to the women's lives (Roberto & Johnston, 1991).

Formal Programs of Support. Many health care professionals provide women with limited details about their osteoporosis. They tend to focus primarily on what the women should not do rather than on what they *can* do to maintain a healthy lifestyle. Older women must be assertive and ask for more specific information about their osteoporosis that will help them make informed decisions about their treatment options. Having accurate and up-to-date knowledge of the disease process also provides older women the opportunity to modify their lifestyles and cope more effectively with the potential consequences of their disease.

Education provided by physicians and other members of the health care team is an essential component of the total treatment plan for women with osteoporosis. Older women need to understand the disease process and what they can do to guard against further deterioration. For example, intermittent ERT is not adequate for preventing postmenopausal bone loss. Yet, noncompliance rates among postmenopausal women using ERT range from 25 to 75 percent (Nachtigall, 1990; Ravnikar, 1987). Physicians need to explain thoroughly the benefits, side effects, and required regime of ERT so that older women have a better understanding of what to expect from this type of intervention.

Participation in more structured programs also help older women better cope and adapt to their osteoporosis. Formal educational programs, such as the Duke University Prevention and Therapeutic Program for Osteoporosis (DUPATPO) provide individuals with factual information about the disease process and help them develop coping skills to physically and emotionally manage their osteoporosis (Gold, Bales, Lyles, & Drezner, 1989). Participants completing this program reported fewer periods of depression, greater potential use of appropriate coping strategies (e.g., inhibition of actions that could be physically or emotionally harmful) and greater comfort in asking for help from others than prior to their participation.

A concerted effort also needs to be made to encourage women at risk for osteoporosis to engage in health promotion strategies aimed at decreasing the likelihood of developing this condition. Patient education and screening programs can be effective in heightening the awareness of targeted individuals and helping women institute behavioral changes in lifestyle conducive to building or sustaining bone mass (Cook, Notelovitz, Rector, & Krischer, 1991; Doyle & Rajacich, 1991).

CONCLUSIONS

With the growth of the elderly population, the number of older women suffering some form of osteoporosis is likely to escalate. Although our understanding of the physiological aspects of osteoporosis has increased significantly over the past decade, scientists must continue to search for a cure and optimal methods of treating and preventing this devastating disease. As part of this process, researchers also must continue their study of the psychosocial consequences of living with osteoporosis and the strategies older women use to maintain healthy and productive lifestyles. Practitioners must encourage women with osteoporosis to continue with their daily activities and social relationships, even though it may require them to change their routines and approach life in new and different ways. As one 78-year old woman asserts, "Having osteoporosis may slow you down a little bit, . . . but you can't just sit and let life pass you over!"

REFERENCES

Albers, M. (1990). Osteoporosis: A health issue for women. *Health Care for Women International, 11,* 11-19.

Bales, C. (1990). Nutritional aspects of osteoporosis: Recommendations for the elderly at risk. In M.P. Lawton (Ed.), *Annual review of gerontology and geriatrics, Vol. 9* (pp. 7-34). New York: Springer.

Bourguet, C., Hamrick, G., & Gilchrist, V. (1991). The prevalence of osteoporosis risk factors and physician intervention. *The Journal of Family Practice, 32,* 265-271.

Cohen, S., & McKay, G. (1984). Social support, stress and the buffering hypothesis: A theoretical analysis. In A. Baun, S. Taylor, & J. Singer (Eds.), *Handbook of psychology and health,* (pp. 253-267). Hillsdale, NJ: Lawrence Erlbaum Associates.

Consensus Conference on Osteoporosis (1984). *Journal of the American Medical Association, 252,* 799-802.

Cook, B., Notelovitz, M., Rector, C., & Krischer, J. (1991). An osteoporosis patient education and screening program: Results and implications. *Patient Education and Counseling, 17,* 134-145.

Department of Health and Human Services. (1991). *Osteoporosis research, education and health promotion.* Washington, DC: National Institutes of Health.

Doyle, R., & Rajacich, D. (1991). The Roy adaptation model: Health teaching about osteoporosis. *AAOHN Journal, 39,* 508-512.

Dupont, W., & Page, D. (1991). Menopausal estrogen replacement therapy and breast cancer. *Archives of Internal Medicine, 151,* 67-72.

Eriksen, E., Hodgson, S., & Riggs, B. L. (1988). Treatment of osteoporosis with sodium fluoride. In B. L. Riggs & L.J. Melton (Eds.), *Osteoporosis etiology, diagnosis, and management* (pp. 373-388). New York: Raven.

Fujita, T. (1992). Vitamin D in the treatment of osteoporosis. *Proceedings of the Society for Experimental Biology and Medicine, 199,* 394-399.

Genant, H., Baylink, D., & Gallagher, J. (1989). Estrogens in the prevention of osteoporosis in postmenopausal women. *American Journal of Obstetrics & Gynecology, 161,* 1842-1849.

Gold, D., Bales, C., Lyles, K., & Drezner, M. (1989). Treatment of osteoporosis: The psychological impact of a medical education program on older patients. *Journal of the American Geriatrics Society, 37,* 417-422.

Gold, D., Lyles, K., Bales, C., & Drezner, M. (1989). Teaching patients coping behaviors: An essential part of successful management of osteoporosis. *Journal of Bone and Mineral Research, 4,* 799-801.

Gossel, T. (1991). Calcium supplements. *U.S. Pharmacist, 16,* 26-32.

Gutin, B., & Kasper, M. (1992). Can vigorous exercise play a role in osteoporosis prevention? A review. *Osteoporosis International, 2,* 55-69.

Hallal, J. (1991). Back pain with postmenopausal osteoporosis and vertebral fractures. *Geriatric Nursing, 12,* 285-287.

Heidrich, F., & Thompson, R. (1987). Osteoporosis prevention: Strategies applicable for general population groups. *The Journal of Family Practice, 25,* 33-39.

Licata, A. (1991). Current treatment modalities for osteoporosis. *Pharmacy Times, 57,* 57-61.

Lufkin, E., Wahner, H., O'Fallon, W., Hodgson, S., Kotowicz, M., Lane, A., Judd, H., Caplan, R., & Riggs, L. (1992). Treatment of postmenopausal osteoporosis with transdermal estrogen. *Annals of Internal Medicine, 117,* 1-9.

McIlwain, H., Fulghum, B., Silverfield, J., & Burnette, M. (1988). *Osteoporosis: Prevention, management, and treatment.* New York: John Wiley & Sons.

McKeon, V. (1990). Estrogen replacement therapy: Current guidelines for education and counseling. *Journal of Gerontological Nursing, 16,* 6-11.

Miller, P. (1992). A guide to the management of osteoporosis and prevention of hip fracture in women. *Modern Medicine, 60,* 46-52.

Munnings, F. (1992). Osteoporosis: What is the role of exercise? *The Physician and Sports Medicine, 20,* 127-138.

Nachtigall, L. (1990). Enhancing patient compliance with hormone replacement therapy at menopause. *Obstetrics and Gynecology, 75,* 77S-80S.

National Osteoporosis Foundation (1991). *Boning up on osteoporosis: A guide to prevention and treatment.* Washington, DC: National Osteoporosis Foundation.

Notelovitz, M., & Ware, M. (1985). *Stand tall!: Every woman's guide to preventing osteoporosis.* New York: Bantam Books.

Quigley, M., Martin, P., Burnier, A., & Brooks, P. (1987). Estrogen therapy arrests bone loss in elderly women. *American Journal of Obstetrics & Gynecology, 156,* 1516-1523.

Ramazzotto, L., Curro, F., Gates, P., & Paterson, J. (1986). Calcium nutrition and the aging process: A review. *Gerodontology, 5,* 159-168.

Ravnikar, V. (1987). Compliance with hormone therapy. *American Journal of Obstetrics & Gynecology, 156,* 1332-1334.

Riggs, B.L., Hodgson, S., O'Fallon, M., Chao, E., Wahner, H., Muhs, J., Cedel, S., & Melton, L.J. (1990). Effect of fluoride treatment on the fracture rate in postmenopausal women with osteoporosis. *The New England Journal of Medicine, 322,* 802-809.

Riggs, B.L., & Melton, L.J. (1986). Involutional osteoporosis. *The New England Journal of Medicine, 314,* 1676-1686.

Roberto, K. (1988). Women with osteoporosis: The role of the family and service community. *The Gerontologist, 28,* 224-228.

Roberto, K. (1989). Stress and adaptation patterns of older osteoporotic women. *Women and Health, 14,* 105-119.

Roberto, K. (1990). Adjusting to chronic disease: The osteoporotic woman. *Journal of Women & Aging, 2,* 33-47.

Roberto, K., & Johnston, M. (1991). The impact of osteoporosis on the quality of informal relationships. *Journal of Gerontological Social Work, 16,* 179-193.

Roberto, K., & McGraw, S. (1991). Self-perceptions of older women with osteoporosis. *Journal of Women & Aging, 3,* 59-70.

Sagraves, R. (1991). Prevention of osteoporosis in premenopausal and postmenopausal women. *American Journal of Pharmaceutical Education, 55,* 158-166.

Santora, A. (1987). Role of nutrition and exercise in osteoporosis. *The American Journal of Medicine, 82*(Suppl. 1B), 73-79.

Seeman, E., Hopper, J., Bach, L., Cooper, M., Parkinson, E., McKay, J., & Jerums, G. (1989). Reduced bone mass in daughters of women with osteoporosis. *The New England Journal of Medicine, 320,* 554-558.

Shangold, M. (1990). Exercise in the menopausal woman. *Obstetrics and Gynecology, 75,* 53S-58S.

Smith, R. (1992). Osteoporosis. In J. George & S. Ebrahim (Eds.), *Health care for older women.* Oxford: Oxford University Press.

Steinberg, K., Thacker, S., Smith, J., Stroup, D., Zack, M., Flanders, D., Berkelman, R. (1991). A meta-analysis of the effect of estrogen replacement therapy on the risk of breast cancer. *Journal of the American Medical Association, 265,* 1985-1990.

Stevenson, J., Anst, M., Gangar, K., Hillard, T., Lees, B., & Whitehead, M. (1990). Effect of transdermal versus oral hormone replacement therapy on bone density in spine and proximal femur in postmenopausal women. *Lancet, 336,* 265-268.

Whitcroft, S., & Stevenson, J. (1992). Hormone replacement therapy: Risks and benefits. *Clinical Endocrinology, 36,* 15-20.

Living Productively with Arthritis

J. Dianne Garner, DSW
Cheryl H. Kinderknecht, ACSW, LMSW

SUMMARY. Arthritis is the most commonly experienced chronic disease among older women. As such, it is essential for professionals to understand the disease process, treatment options, physiological and psychosocial implications as well as how to assist older arthrictic women in developing and implementing strategies for productive living. The disease process, treatment options, physiological and psychosocial implications are presented. The importance of patient education is stressed in addition to mechanisms for assisting older women in coping with pain, preventing or combating learned helplessness, minimizing functional limitations, addressing issues of sexual functioning, complying with medical regimen, and enhancing social supports. Managing stress and dealing with feelings are also discussed.

Arthritis is a group of diseases characterized by stiffness, chronic pain and loss of movement. Various forms of arthritis affect one-in-seven individuals, or an estimated 37 million Americans, and about half of all Americans over age 65 are affected by arthritis. Although there are over 100 different forms of arthritis, the two most common forms are osteoarthritis and rheumatoid arthritis. Osteoarthritis affects

J. Dianne Garner is Professor and Chair, Department of Social Work at Washburn University, Topeka, KS.
Cheryl H. Kinderknecht is Administrative Officer, Behavioral Sciences Regulatory Board, Topeka, KS.

[Haworth co-indexing entry note]: "Living Productively with Arthritis." Garner, J. Dianne, and Cheryl H. Kinderknecht. Co-published simultaneously in the *Journal of Women & Aging* (The Haworth Press, Inc.) Vol. 5, No. 3/4, 1993, pp. 61-82; and: *Women and Healthy Aging: Living Productively in Spite of It All* (ed: J. Dianne Garner, and Alice A. Young), The Haworth Press, Inc., 1993, pp. 61-82. Multiple copies of this article/chapter may be purchased from The Haworth Document Delivery Center. [1-800-3-HAWORTH; 9:00 a.m.-5:00 p.m. (EST)].

about 16 million Americans (Task Force for Aging Research Funding [TFARF] 1992), the majority of whom are women. Rheumatoid arthritis affects approximately 8 million Americans (Arthritis Foundation, 1986) and occurs two to three times more often in women than men (Bennet, 1985).

Known as the number one crippling disease in America, arthritis is the most widespread and disabling of any of the chronic afflictions affecting humankind (Lambert & Lambert, 1987). The impact of arthritis on individuals and society in terms of physical, emotional, and financial suffering is enormous (TFARF, 1992). Arthritis victims are often faced with incurable chronic pain and the unpredictability of a disease that frequently compromises their quality of life.

DISEASE PROCESS

Osteoarthritis (OA) is a degenerative joint disease characterized by mechanical alterations in the joint, and is often called a "wear-and-tear" disease. Large weight-bearing joints, such as knees and hips, are the sites most often affected, although the spine, ankles, and small joints of the fingers are commonly involved as well. Joint cartilage covers the ends of bones within a joint, serving as both a shock absorber and a load-bearing surface to permit smooth, almost frictionless movement. OA leads to the gradual and insidious deterioration of this protective cartilage. Initially, the smooth surface of the joint cartilage becomes softened, pitted and frayed. With the breakdown of cartilage, some inflammation occurs, although this is usually much less pronounced in OA than in other common forms of arthritis such as rheumatoid arthritis and gout. Gradually, areas of cartilage may be worn away completely, leaving bone to rub on bone. Bony spurs sometimes form at the margins of the joint, where ligaments and the joint capsule are attached. As the OA process continues, the normal shape and mechanical function of the joint are altered.

Rheumatoid arthritis (RA) is a systemic connective tissue disorder of unknown cause in which symptoms and inflammatory changes predominate in joints and related structures. RA and the related rheumatic diseases tend to be chronic, characterized by remissions and exacerbations, and ultimately may produce severely crippling deformities (Bennet, 1985). Symptoms generally begin as generalized fatigue, soreness, stiffness (particularly on rising in the morning), and aching, Localized inflammatory symptoms occur in the affected joints, including pain, swelling, radiating warmth and tenderness. While the inflammatory changes initially occur in the synovial membranes of the joint, outgrowths of the inflamed tissue invade the cartilage that surrounds the bone ends. The resultant soft tissue scarring and bone erosion cause the involved joints to become fragile, permanently rigid and immovable. Persistent inflammation of the joint space can lead to distortion and limiting deformities of the joint. This process of distortion and deformity becomes most apparent when rheumatoid arthritis involves the hands.

Despite its prevalence and destructive nature, knowledge of the etiology and pathogenesis of RA is limited. One of the most widely accepted theories postulates that causality is related to immune factors. According to current beliefs, an unidentified antigen stimulus induces antibody production by the plasma cells in the synovial membrane which secretes the protective, friction-reducing transparent fluid found in joint cavities, bursa and tendon sheaths.

Other common arthritis-related disorders include gout, psoriatic arthritis and ankylosing spondylitis. Gout is an acute, recurrent and potentially chronic and deforming type of arthritis which affects the peripheral joints. Because of high concentrations of uric acid, deposits of monosodium urate cluster in and about the joints and tendons, causing inflammation, swelling, warmth and exquisite tenderness. Psoriatic arthritis is a rheumatoid-like arthritis associated with psoriasis of the skin or nails, in addition to the processes customarily seen in rheumatoid arthritis. Ankylosing spondylitis is a systemic rheumatic disorder characterized primarily by inflammation of the axial skeleton and large peripheral joints.

TREATMENT

Although arthritis is not curable, its symptoms can, in most cases, be alleviated, joint function can be improved and disability can be prevented or reduced. Treatment is generally composed of a combination of joint protection, exercise, medication, heat and cold treatments, weight control and, when necessary, surgery.

Joint protection includes the reduction of stresses and strains to affected joints to prevent increased pain or further damage. Avoidance of activities such as jogging, high-impact aerobics or other activities which result in increased pain is advised. Canes, crutches and walkers may be used to reduce the stress on weight-bearing joints, and upper extremity adaptive devices such as splints and elastic supports can reduce joint stress and provide increased joint stability. Other methods of joint protection include using a firm mattress or bed board, sitting in straight-backed chairs which have arm rests, avoiding sitting for long periods of time and limiting lifting as much as possible.

Regular, appropriate exercise is extremely important in the management of arthritis. Failure to use joints can result in stiffness, reduced mobility and the muscles which provide necessary joint support can become weakened. Exercises such as swimming, walking and pedaling a stationary bicycle are less stressful on joints and are good for overall fitness. Specific active and passive exercises may be prescribed to prevent muscle atrophy and to maintain range of motion of joints.

Nonsteroidal anti-inflammatory drugs, NSAIDS (pronounced en-seds) include aspirin and aspirin-like pain-relieving drugs which help reduce joint pain, stiffness and swelling. Corticosteroids are similar to cortisone, a natural body hormone. Corticosteroids come in pill form, not used for the treatment of osteoarthritis, or may be injected into the joint to relieve pain and the swelling that sometimes occurs with osteoarthritis. Since arthritis is a chronic disease which is not life-threatening, medication with high levels of toxicity are generally avoided. Unfortunately, the drugs of choice in the treatment of arthritis can have multiple side-effects, including epigastric distress, nausea and gastrointestinal bleeding. However, taking coated anti-inflammatory drugs or taking medication with meals may alleviate or prevent some side effects.

Heat and cold treatments are effective ways to temporarily relieve pain and soreness. A hot bath or shower just after getting out of bed may relieve the pain and stiffness frequently experienced after sleep. Hot packs, heat lamps, moist electric heating pads, electric mitts and paraffin wax are also methods of using heat to relieve joint pain and stiffness. Cold treatments, such as cold compresses or ice cubes wrapped in towels can numb the area resulting in lessening of the pain sensation.

Weight control is an important element in the treatment of arthritis. Extra pounds put even more stress on weight-bearing joints. This extra stress can lead to further joint pain and damage. Losing weight can also result in increased energy and feeling healthier in general.

Particularly in advanced rheumatoid arthritis and advanced cases of osteoarthritis, surgery may be indicated. Severely damaged joints may be replaced or repaired surgically with wear-resistant artificial joints. Total hip and knee replacements have been used for a longer time than other joint replacement procedures, and are among the most successful. Less dramatic surgical procedures may be needed to remove damaged tissue and clear the way for smooth movement. As a general rule, surgery produces the best results when balanced with medications and a program of physical activity (Arthritis Foundation, 1990).

Many arthritis patients commonly utilize nontraditional treatment modalities while continuing to employ standard health care practices. Surveys indicate that anywhere from one-third to over 90% of arthritis patients turn to nontraditional treatments. Commonly used practices include unusual diets, wearing a copper bracelet, vitamins, folk remedies and acupuncture. Other treatments tried with less frequency include cod liver oil, alfalfa, yucca, sea water, vaccines, Mexican "cures" and uranium. While some of these 'treatments' are essentially harmless, others, such as steroid or hormone vaccinations, are potentially quite dangerous, frequently expensive and of no proven value (Arthritis Foundation, 1983).

PHYSIOLOGICAL IMPACTS

Clinical features of arthritis include pain in the affected joints, particularly with motion and weight bearing, and a stiffening sensation is common after periods of rest. Spasm and atrophy of muscles surrounding the diseased joint are common. The joint enlarges as a result of the bony swelling, accumulation of fluid, thickening of or damage to the soft tissue and, ultimately, motion of the joint becomes limited. Patients with knee and hip involvement are sometimes unable to ambulate. Those with hand involvement may suffer crippling deformities resulting in hands which are difficult to use properly when performing common activities of daily living such as grooming, using kitchen utensils, dialing the telephone or writing. Fatigue is a frequent and troubling symptom of many forms of arthritis, particularly those which affect the whole body such as rheumatoid arthritis (Arthritis Foundation, 1991).

The usual course of the arthritis is one of persistent progression punctuated by remissions and acute exacerbations of the inflammatory process (Lambert, Lambert, Klipple & Mewshaw, 1989). In mild cases, functional impairment is confined to pain and modest limitations during acute phases. In severe cases, there is chronic pain coupled with marked bony deformity and limitation of motion. The patient may be confined to a wheelchair, to her home or she may be completely bedfast and totally dependent on others for care. Mechanical limitations may also impose significant obstacles to sexual functioning. For example, a woman with severe arthritis of the hip joints may be unable to spread her legs wide enough for sexual intercourse in the standard frontal position, or the weight of her partner's body may produce severe pain. The degree of functional limitation depends on both the amount of mobility restriction experienced and the degree of joint pain encountered.

Particularly in the case of RA, there is a likelihood of severe impairment due to the insidious crippling nature of the disease. In a longitudinal study of the disease's effects, it was found that at the end of 20 years, 54% of the subjects were either dead or severely disabled despite aggressive treatment (Scott, Symmons, Coulton & Popert, 1987). Although medical regimens can positively influence the short term and medium term prognoses, the long term outlook for many RA patients is still poor. Since adult onset RA typically begins in mid life, it is during the later years that women are experiencing its most painful and crippling effects.

Arthritis is a painful disease involving both acute and chronic pain of variable intensity. Acute arthritic pain occurs during periods of disease flare-ups and exacerbation or when affected joints are overused. Acute pain is characterized by new inflammation and tissue damage, anxiety and observable changes in respiration, blood pressure and heart rate. Acute pain generally subsides as the flare-up subsides and the body becomes accustomed to the changes. Chronic pain is ever present and the persistent sensation of pain may result in the unnecessary avoidance of virtually all activity. However, overuse of a chronically painful joint may result in acute pain and/or further damage. Finding the delicate and individualized balance between exercise which will strengthen and protect chronically affected joints and that which will result in acute pain or further damage poses a challenge for professionals and patients alike.

PSYCHOSOCIAL IMPLICATIONS

Arthritis has important psychosocial implications which need to be understood and addressed by health care providers. Because in the early stages, arthritis is not a visible illness and many people still consider arthritis a minor disease, lack of understanding and support can be problematic for older women with arthritis and can further complicate psychosocial adjustment.

Often causing major changes in life-style, arthritis imposes a wide variety of losses on its victims, including varying degrees of loss of mobility, loss of function, loss of independence and loss of customary roles and relationships. The arthritic's emotional responses to these losses are similar to those of terminally ill patients (Gross, 1981). Kubler-Ross (1969) identified five stages within the emotional response of terminally ill patients: denial, anger, bargaining, depression and acceptance. Because arthritis is characterized by periods of exacerbation and remission, there is frequently back and forth movement and repetition of these emotional response stages.

The nature and severity of arthritis directly influence the psychological well-being of individuals who are forced to contend with this chronic and disabling illness. Self-reports of depression are common among arthritis patients, regardless of the type of arthritis that is involved. Lower levels of self-esteem and increased feelings of meaninglessness were also found among RA patients (Bradley, 1985). In addition, Burckhardt (1985) found arthritis sufferers who were depressed, discouraged, angry, worried or frustrated about their disease experienced a lower quality of life.

Research findings have consistently demonstrated that the occurrence of stressful events can lead to an exacerbation of symptoms in the arthritic and/or to an increased incidence in the development of stress-related illnesses. Stress increases physiological responses such as the production of adrenal cortical and adrenal medullary hormones. These increased levels of natural corticosteroids can result in decreased immunologic responses which, in turn, can lead to a lowered body resistance and an increased susceptibility to the development of some illnesses (Lambert & Lambert, 1987).

Professional literature focusing on arthritis reveals recurrent psychosocial themes. These themes include responses to pain, locus of control and learned helplessness, responses to functional limitations and psychosexual issues. Also included are the issues relating to treatment compliance and the patient's social support system.

In contrast to the traditional belief that pain is a purely biological phenomenon, it is a complex phenomenon that involves physiological, psychological and social components. Two primary psychological characteristics are common among people with chronic pain: depression, because life is disrupted on many levels, and low self-esteem, because patients feel useless and ineffective (Montague & Stein, 1989). The literature suggests that self-reports of pain among arthritics are positively correlated with self-reports of depression and that patients' self-reports of pain are more important than physical or psychological disability in explaining medication usage (Kazis, Meenan & Anderson, 1983). In addition, the desire to hide her pain or to prevent others from witnessing her pain can lead to self-imposed isolation from friends and family.

A persistent perception of external control (or lack of personal control) can lead to the learned helplessness, a behavior pattern characterized by pervasive feelings of helplessness resulting from the belief that outcomes are not influenced by one's own actions (Seligman, 1975). The behavior pattern of learned helplessness is generally characterized by emotional, cognitive and motivational deficits in coping with stressful situations. For the arthritic patient, learned helplessness is found to be associated with high levels of pain, anxiety and depression, low self-esteem and low satisfaction with current functional abilities (Bradley, 1985). Uncertainties connected with pain, prognosis and long-term functional implications contribute to a sense of helplessness and loss of control for the arthritis patient. The added anxiety of not knowing the problems with which one will have to cope increases the feelings of helplessness.

The literature indicates that patients with RA may be particularly likely to develop the belief that their disease is beyond their effective control because the cause and cure for the disease are unknown and the course and final outcomes of the disease are unpredictable. Bradley (1985) points out that studies involving RA patients' attitudes reveal that perceptions of helplessness are indeed associated with increased disease activity or increased functional impairment.

Burckhardt (1985) demonstrated that the higher the severity of impairment, the lower one's self-esteem and perception of quality of life. The extent of functional impairment negatively impacts on life satisfaction, as well as directly influencing the amount of restriction of physical activity. The inability to participate in once enjoyable activities may then lead to social isolation and depression. Older women suffering from moderate to severe arthritis may require several hours daily to complete self-care activities and are frequently unwilling to freely admit to the difficulty or to ask for assistance.

The psychological and physiological impact of arthritis has significant implications on intimacy. Deyo et al. (1982) found that 46% of RA patients reported decreased sexual activity since disease onset. Manne and Zautra (1989) found that husbands were often critical of their wives in regard to the limitations her illness imposed on their sexual activities. A greater incidence of divorce and a lower rate of remarriage was found among female RA patients and the lower rate of remarriage following divorce was specifically attributed to the course of the disease.

A variety of sexual concerns appear to be very common among arthritis patients. Often, sexual activity is inhibited by the presence or threat of physical pain. Underlying feelings of depression and low self-esteem frequently experienced by individuals with chronic illnesses can impede the libido. Body image, particularly among individuals with deforming arthritis, may also present a barrier to sexuality and intimacy. The degree of interference of body image with sexual functioning has been found to depend on the prior pattern of adaptation, the extent of body changes or limitations and the emotional value the patient attaches to the body part or function

(Campbell, 1984). Immobility or partial mobility of joints can result in decreased sexual activity and, when mobility difficulties are accompanied by pain, can result in total abstinence particularly when there is lack of knowledge regarding alternate positions or lack of willingness to explore options. In actuality, any of the factors listed or combination of factors, may result in total loss of sexual intimacy. In addition, older women are frequently facing body image adjustments secondary to the process of aging and may be dealing with loss of intimacy secondary to death of a spouse or divorce.

Arthritis patients are consistently shown to vary widely with regard to compliance with medication regimen, physical therapy instructions and splint use. Factors predictive on nonadherence include disease severity and duration of illness with more severe and longer term patients less likely to be compliant (Bradley, 1985). Patients who were once compliant may begin to feel hopeless or to seek costly and potentially dangerous nontraditional treatments as medical regimens fail to "cure" the disease.

Aversive factors associated with arthritis include severe pain, progressive deterioration and deformity, disease flare-ups, dependency on others and threats to both self-image and esteem. To successfully adapt to the many demands of the disease process, arthritis patients may have a greater than average need for social supports (Manne & Zautra, 1989). Social support is defined as the interpersonal transaction that involves the expression of affection toward another; the endorsement or affirmation of another's behavior, perceptions or views; and the giving of material, symbolic or concrete aid to another (Kahn, 1979). Social support can modify the negative effects of stressful situations such as chronic illness either by reducing stress or by facilitating the individual's ability to cope with the stress. Historical and current studies have produced clear evidence that patients' reports of effective coping and low levels of psychological distress are associated with high levels of perceived social support (Bradley, 1985). The greater the social support that an individual receives in the form of close relationships, the more likely it is that the negative aspects of illness and disability will be buffered (Burckhardt, 1985).

In responding to the patient's disease, family members also experience a variety of emotional reactions. The reactions of family members may commonly include denial, anger and depression. Therefore, presence of family members does not necessarily translate into support.

While studies suggest that there is no remarkable difference in the social support characteristics between ethnic groups, arthritis patients of higher socioeconomic groups and those who are married appear to have more sources and types of support available to them (Lambert & Lambert, 1985). Manne and Zautra (1989) found that patient adjustment is significantly related to the attitude of the spouse. Patients with a highly critical spouse engaged in more maladaptive coping behaviors and reported a poorer psychological adjustment than did those patients who perceived their spouse as being supportive. Empirical studies clearly indicate that satisfaction with social support is a significant predictor of psychosocial well-being (Lambert, Lambert, Klipple & Mewshaw, 1989).

STRATEGIES FOR PRODUCTIVE LIVING

While arthritis is a disease of all age groups and both sexes, it disproportionately affects older women. The combination of acute and chronic pain coupled with joint stiffness and immobility can result in activity limitations from basic, daily activities such as dressing oneself to recreational and social outlets such as dancing. Older women with arthritis are challenged daily to learn to do things differently and/or to do different things. Subtle and radical changes are frequently necessary, depending on the disease severity and the life style of the older woman with arthritis. For example: the 75-year old woman who has already been swimming regularly at the 'Y' may find no need to alter that activity, while the sedentary 75-year old woman will need to begin an alien process of routine, low impact exercise, and the 75-year old woman who plays tennis will need to find substitute appropriate exercises. Given the multiple changes and adaptations necessary for arthritic older women, assistance in making adaptations must come from a variety of professional disciplines.

While almost every arthritis patient will have the need for professional support in addition to the "hands on" medical treatment, the degree of assistance needed to attain the goal of living productively with arthritis will be highly individualized. Many older women will already possess good coping skills, have intact social supports, be actively involved with community and/or family and will make adjustments and adaptations which enable them to continue to live and age productively with, or in spite of, arthritis and with minimal professional assistance. Others will need assistance in developing coping skills and may, for a variety of reasons, rely heavily on professionals in assisting with their adaptation.

An important initial step in assisting older women in maintaining a satisfying quality of life is getting to know the individual. Examples of questions that need to be asked and answered are as follows: What activities does she find enjoyable? How has she coped with adversity in the past? What natural supports does she have? What are her financial and insurance resources? What does she view as her roles and responsibilities? What does she know and understand about her disease and its treatment? How does she feel about her disease? What does she see as the limitations arthritis imposes on her life? It is important to note that older women have as many differences as do younger age cohorts. Myths and stereotypes about old women must be discarded and replaced by accurate and thorough information regarding each individual. Not only will the type of disease, disease severity and course of illness vary widely among individual older women, but responses to the disease will vary widely. Once sufficient information is obtained about the individual, strategies for enhancing productive living in the older arthritic woman include educating her about her disease, assisting her with pain management and coping with pain, helping her prevent or combat learned helplessness, assisting her in minimizing functional limitations, addressing problems of sexual functioning, helping her comply with prescribed treatments, and assisting her in enhancing social supports.

Educating

In order to adapt to any illness, it is important for the individual to understand the disease and its consequences. She needs to know that arthritis is chronic and that there is no "cure." She needs to understand that symptoms and progression can be managed and that she is a central player in the management of her disease. Treatments need to be fully explained, including both benefits and possible side effects.

Although the course of arthritis can be unpredictable, reasonable perimeters regarding the course of her illness should be explained. The purpose of assistive devices and how to use them should be outlined in detail. When needed assistive devices are not affordable and not available at reduced or no cost through a community agency, information regarding how to make a device should be given. For example: a back-scratcher from K-Mart can extend reaching ability and two back-scratchers connected by rubber bands using a small block of wood as a fulcrum makes a crude but effective reacher with the ability to grasp some objects. Many professionals have learned from arthritics useful inexpensive adaptive mechanisms which should be shared, as appropriate, with other arthritis victims.

Professionals must be aware that patient education is an ongoing process. Not only do situations change, but both newly diagnosed arthritics and arthritics experiencing new disease developments are likely to respond initially with denial or anger which may well block their ability to process information. Therefore, information relative to new developments and information previously given to newly diagnosed arthritics may need to be repeated at intervals. In addition, asking the patient to repeat back information she has been given increases the likelihood of retention.

There are multiple pamphlets and educational booklets available at no cost through organizations such as the Arthritis Foundation. Easily understandable printed material, when given to the patient, has the additional benefit of being able to be read repeatedly and at her leisure. For older women who have vision difficulties, printed material will need to be available with large, black, block lettering on non-gloss white paper. Educational cassettes are also available for older women whose vision precludes the use of printed material. Whatever methods or combination of methods are used in educating arthritics, education is imperative to the adaptive process. The reality is that only a knowledgeable patient is able to make rational decisions regarding her illness, participate in the process of managing her illness and hence make the necessary adaptations for a productive and satisfying life.

Managing or Coping with Pain

Assisting patients in assuming control over their pain has the potential to positively enhance their coping ability and their perceptions of their quality of life. In addition to the use of medications, there are several means of actively assisting patients in learning to control their pain.

Gate theory. When there is an injury or inflammation, the injury site sends a message to the brain through a mechanism that works like a gate (Montague & Stein, 1989). Physical, emotional and cognitive factors can open or close the gate. For example: joint strain or misuse, emotional upset or negative thoughts can open the gate, releasing sensations of pain while medication, appropriate exercise, positive thoughts, involvement and a sense of personal control can close the gate, limiting the perception of pain.

Muscle relaxation. Muscle tension and spasms frequently accompany pain. As the arthritic experiences pain, muscles in the surrounding area become rigid or tense and may spasm, increasing the perception of pain. Relaxation exercises, guided imagery and stress reduction activities can reduce muscle tension and diminish pain. Bradley, Young, Anderson et al. (1987) found that arthritis patients consistently identified relaxation and imagery training as one of the most helpful components of treatment.

Cognitive therapy. Based on the theory that affect and behavior are largely influenced by thoughts and beliefs, cognitive therapy is designed to help patients identify and correct distorted or dysfunctional beliefs. By listening carefully it is possible for professionals to identify negative thoughts and beliefs which influence the actions or inactions of the arthritis patient. Supportive, rather than confrontational, assistance helps her identify, modify or eliminate negative thoughts and beliefs which tend to contribute to or magnify the sensation of pain.

Other effective pain management mechanisms usually include multiple components such as education, coping skills training and praise for appropriate coping behavior. Most importantly, arthritis "patients are encouraged to take responsibility for managing their pain and disabilities with their newly learned skills and to attribute successes to their own actions" (Bradley, 1985, p. 8).

Preventing or Combating Learned Helplessness

To prevent or combat learned helplessness, it is imperative for professionals to assist the patient in the realization that she does have some control over the stressful life situations caused by her arthritis. Which coping mechanisms she uses, how and when coping mechanisms are used and how effective her coping mechanisms are must be determined so that appropriate remedial actions can be planned and implemented. Taking time to explain the disease process and treatment plan may increase understanding of the disease and lead to feelings of increased internal control over both health and quality of life. To increase the patient's sense of predictability, it is important to help her recognize that there will be good days and bad days. Having accurate information about such factors as what intensifies and contributes to arthritic pain, what alterations or modifications of life style enhance functioning and what community agencies are available for assistance can contribute to her perception of control over her situation.

Assisting the patient in understanding the causal relationship between her efforts and managing her arthritis is critical in preventing and combating feelings of helplessness. Provision of, or referral to, assertiveness training programs and advocacy groups will further reinforce a sense of control as will actively involving the patient in decisions regarding her own care and treatment.

Minimizing Functional Limitations

In order to assist the patient in minimizing functional limitations, functional limitations must first be assessed. Obtaining a detailed account of the arthritic older woman's customary day, including reports of pain and difficulty in accomplishing activities, is most helpful in assessing functional limitations. This information may reveal that special adaptive equipment, such as a long-handled bathbrush, comb or 'reacher' will allow her to be more independent. Adaptive clothing with velcro fasteners–rather than buttons, zippers and snaps–might reduce the time, effort and pain involved in getting dressed. Her account of a customary day may indicate the need for environmental modifications to optimize functioning and independence such as installing grab bars next to the toilet and bathtub, having ramps installed and elevating straight-backed armchairs and the bed 3 or 4 inches. If there appear to be unmet needs for adaptive devices or environmental modifications, an occupational therapist can be very helpful. Specially trained to evaluate and maximize functional independence, the occupational therapist is a vital member of the arthritis health care team. Similarly, a physical therapist can offer invaluable assistance with such activities as helping the patient maximize mobility and major joint function and educating her on how to protect against joint strain and injury.

Community agencies offer a variety of services which can assist in minimizing the effects of functional limitations. Home health care, home delivered meals and homemaker/chore services are particularly helpful when completion of basic self-care or household tasks is problematic. Low or no cost assistive devices, transportation, medical assistance or appropriate housing may be available through community agencies. Linking the patient to the resources and services that optimize functioning, reduce dependency and alleviate stress all tend to enhance the patient's sense of personal control and well-being as well as maximizing her functional independence.

Addressing Problems of Sexual Functioning

In order to effectively address sexual concerns, professionals need to convey an open, accepting and nonjudgemental attitude toward both the older woman and the topic. Unfortunately, health care workers have been reluctant to bring up sexual concerns, particularly with the aged. This reluctance appears to reflect our society's tendency to 'neuter' the elderly even though professional literature consistently indicates that human beings can and do remain sexually active throughout old age. Cessation of sexual activity in old age is most often related to loss of a partner or to diseases, such as arthritis, which can inhibit sexual functioning. The absence of a wedding ring does not necessarily indicate there is no partner and does not absolve the professional from addressing sexual concerns. A single older woman may be involved in a dating relationship or living with a partner. Even if the older woman is without a partner, she may have sexual concerns for a future date. The first challenge for professionals in assisting older arthritic women with sexual functioning is the willingness to recognize older women as sexual beings. Once that hurdle is overcome, information about sexual functioning with arthritis is applicable.

Although patients may initially deny that they have questions or concerns about sexual functioning, introducing the subject may give the patient or her partner permission to bring up sexual matters at a later time. Without an opening from a health care professional the older woman may mistakenly assume she is barred for life from sexual intimacy because of her arthritis.

In addition to supportive counseling relating to intimacy and sexuality, professionals who work with arthritics should be able to provide education about sexual matters and adaptations that specifically pertain to the arthritis patient. This may include verbal information or literature relating to preparation for sexual activity, alternate positions for intercourse, and other possible ways of expressing sexual feelings. In addition, changes in body image secondary to both aging and arthritis should be discussed.

Professionals who are uncomfortable in discussing sexuality with older women should identify someone on the health care team who is willing and able to assume that role. Another option is to leave literature out and readily available for arthritic patients to read and/or take home with them. However, it should be recognized that literature alone does not afford the patient the opportunity to ask questions. It should also be recognized that supportive, intimate relationships positively impact on self-esteem and perceived quality of life, including those among older women.

Assisting with Compliance

Protecting joints through avoiding activities such as jogging or excessive lifting; regular, appropriate exercise to increase or maintain mobility, decrease pain, and strengthen surrounding muscles; use of medication to reduce inflammation; swelling and pain; weight control to reduce stress on joints; and hot and cold packs to reduce pain, are all a part of treating or managing arthritis. Patient education which includes supportive and practical instructions on the benefits of following treatment regimen has been shown to have a significant impact on compliance (Lorig, Konkol & Gonzales, 1987). Easy-to-open prescription bottles enhance medication compliance among arthritics with hand involvement. Individualizing treatment plans which capitalize on the patient's strengths and adaptive coping skills enhance feelings of internal control and make compliance more likely. Allowing the patient to participate in decisions about management of her disease also increases the likelihood of compliance.

Having the patient keep a daily journal detailing when medication was taken and the exercise program was carried out can assist in assessing compliance and patient understanding of the regimen as prescribed. It also involves her in the management of her treatment, increasing probable compliance, and the act of keeping a journal may help remind and motivate her toward compliance. If the patient is instructed to record the times and precipitating factors when intense pain is experienced, it may assist in making adaptations which decrease intense pain, hence increase compliance. It is also possible that including intensely experienced pain in the journal may have a cathartic effect for the arthritis patient, allowing her a safe and sanctioned place to express pain.

Enhancing Social Supports

While the majority of older women live in families, 42% live alone (AARP, 1992). It is, therefore, necessary to determine who makes up the patient's support network, who provides what support and who provides the most effective and satisfying support. Since the patient's ability to cope appears to be linked to the supportiveness of significant others (Manne & Zautra, 1989), it is important to consider both the positive and negative aspects of social relationships. Upon identifying the strengths and limitations of the immediate support network, it may be necessary to expand the network to include formal sources of support.

Assisting in maintaining the support network is an essential task. Listening to family members, recognizing the legitimacy of their feelings, clarifying concerns or misconceptions, providing emotional support and assisting in obtaining services from community agencies can alleviate the burdens inherent in care giving. In addition, the family should be given specific information relating to the nature and course of arthritis, predictable patient responses to the disease and frequently experienced family reactions. Appropriate adaptive coping mechanisms of family members should be identified and reinforced.

Coordination of informal and formal sources of support is often necessary to ensure that the support network continues to operate smoothly. Use of community services and agencies is not only a benefit to the patient but to her family as well. Obtaining appropriate assistive devices enables the patient to be more independent, places less stress on joints and relieves her family from having to provide assistance with tasks which can be accomplished by the patient with the use of such devices.

Older women who live alone and are socially isolated are at considerable risk for premature or avoidable decline of both physical functioning and psychological well-being. Appropriately networking the isolated woman into formal supportive services is of prime importance in such circumstances. In the absence of informal supports, the informational, educational and emotional support provided by health care professionals and community agency personnel or volunteers can go a long way toward satisfying the social support needs of the isolated arthritic older woman.

Other mechanisms for assisting older women make the necessary adaptations include assisting her in managing stress, appropriately expressing her feelings and appropriately using humor. As previously pointed out both stress and negative feelings exacerbate arthritic flare-ups and the sensation of pain. Stress is a response the body makes when called upon to make too many changes. Arthritis patients may have additional stress related to pain, medical expenses and concerns for the future. Assisting the patient in accepting what she cannot change rather than feeling constantly frustrated will considerably lessen stress (Arthritis Foundation, 1986). Regular exercise, relaxation therapy and biofeedback are also effective in reducing or managing stress. Negative feelings, particularly depression and anger, are normal in the face of changes like those experienced due to arthritis. However, if unexpressed, or expressed inappropriately, they can lead to increased stress and tension and fatigue. Assisting the arthritic in appropriately expressing feelings and use of such techniques such as assertiveness training and relaxation therapy can eliminate or appreciably reduce the consequences of negative emotion. In addition, helping the patient become involved in purposeful, enjoyable activities may result in significant reduction or elimination of depression.

Humor, when used appropriately, can be an effective defense mechanism and a preventative device for avoiding anger, depression or feelings of hopelessness. In recent years, the ability to laugh, even in the most dire of circumstances, has been positively correlated to slowing down the disease process, lessening the sensation of pain and perceived improvement in overall health. However, professionals must be very cautious in the use of humor lest they be perceived as uncaring, unfeeling or making fun of the patient or her situation. Patient support groups are known to increase the appropriate use of humor as arthritics themselves share situations related to their disease in a humorous way.

CONCLUSION

The most frequently occurring chronic condition among the elderly in the United States (Arthritis Foundation, 1992), arthritis is a condition routinely seen by multiple professionals. While the percentage of older women affected by arthritis may remain fixed, the numbers will grow as demographics continue to shift toward increased longevity. The nature and severity of arthritis directly influences the psychosocial well-being of women who are forced to contend with this chronic and disabling illness. The prevalence and nature of arthritis are such that professionals will continue to play a critical role in the care of older women with arthritis and in assisting them in making appropriate adaptations.

At a recent professional meeting in New York, an emeritus professor, who appeared to be in her eighties, riddled with crippling arthritis and ambulating on a walker, was frequently observed participating vigorously in multiple conversations. She had traveled a great distance to be there and, when asked if it wasn't difficult given her illness, she laughed and replied, "As long as I'm busy, I don't even think about my arthritis." She went on to state that the hardest part had been the long plane flight. However, she had kept her mind occupied by working on her next book. Gnarled fingers which probably could not begin to hold a pencil, remained productive using a lap top computer. There was little question that assistive devices were used daily and that velcro substituted for buttons. As we work with older arthritic women, let us remember the aged professor and author whose adaptability, good humor and courage allow her to overcome the adversities of arthritis and continue a productive, fulfilling life.

FIFTIETH HIGH SCHOOL REUNION

As young girls we lusted for clothes, boys
and unblemished skin.
As young mothers we lusted for sleep
and free time alone
As middle aged divorcees and widows
we lusted for men our age
who preferred much younger women.
Now, nearing seventy
We lust for children's phone calls
and arthritis relief.

–Ruth Harriet Jacobs
also published in
Poet Magazine, Summer, 1992

NOTE

For additional information contact: The Arthritis Foundation P.O. Box 19000 Atlanta, GA 30326 1-800-283-7800.

REFERENCES

American Association of Retired Persons (1992). A profile of older Americans, Washington, DC: Author.

Arthritis Foundation (1983). Basic facts: answers to your questions. Atlanta, GA: Author.

Arthritis Foundation (1991). Coping with fatigue. Atlanta, GA: Author.

Arthritis Foundation (1990). Osteoarthritis. Atlanta, GA: Author.

Arthritis Foundation (1986). Taking charge learning to live with arthritis. Atlanta, GA: Author.

Arthritis Foundation, Metropolitan Washington DC Chapter (1986). Fact sheet on arthritis. Arlington, VA: Author.

Bennet, J.C. (1985). Rheumatoid arthritis. In J. Wyugaarden & L. Smith. (eds.) Cecil's Textbook of Medicine. 17th edition. Philadelphia, PA: W.B. Saunders.

Bradley, L.A. (1985). Psychological aspects of arthritis. Arthritis Foundation Bulletin on the Rheumatic Diseases, Vol. 35(4), pp. 1-12.

Bradley, L.A.; Young, L.B.; Anderson, K.O.; Turner, R.A.; Agudelo, C.A.; McDaniel, L.K.; Pisko, E.J.; Semble, E.L., & Morgan, T.M. (1987). Effects of psychological therapy on pain behavior of rheumatoid arthritis patients: treatment outcome and six-month follow-up. Arthritis and Rheumatism, Vol. 30(10), pp. 1105-1114.

Burckhardt, C. (1985). The impact of arthritis on quality of life. Nursing Research, Vol. 34, pp. 11-16.

Campbell, S.J. (1984). Sexuality assessment. In J.P. Bellack & P.A. Bamford (eds.) Nursing assessment: a multidimensional approach, pp. 173-202. Monterey, CA: Wadsworth Health Sciences Division.

Deyo, R.A.; Inui, T.S.; Leininger, J., & Overman, S. (1982). Physical and psychosocial function in rheumatoid arthritis: clinical use of a self-administered health status instrument. Archives of International Medicine, Vol. 142, pp. 879-882.

Gross, M. (1981). Psychosocial aspects of osteoarthritis: helping patients cope. Health & Social Work, Vol. 4, pp. 40-46.

Kahn, R. (1979). Aging and social support. In M.W. Riley (ed.) Aging from birth to death: interdisciplinary perspectives. Boulder, CO: Westview Press.

Kazis, L.E.; Meenan, R.F., & Anderson. J.J. (1983). Pain in the rheumatic diseases. Arthritis and Rheumatism, Vol. 26, pp. 1017-1022.

Kubler-Ross, E. (1969). On death and dying. New York, NY: Macmillan Publishing Co.

Lambert, V.A. & Lambert, C.E. (1987). Coping with rheumatoid arthritis. Nursing Clinics of North America, Vol. 22(3), pp. 551-558.

Lambert, V.A. & Lambert, C.E. (1985). The relationship between social support and psychological well-being in rheumatoid arthritic women from two ethnic groups. Health Care for Women International, Vol. 6, pp. 405-414.

Lambert, V.A.; Lambert, C.E.; Klipple, G.L., & Mewshaw, E.A. (1989). Social support, hardiness and psychological well-being in women with arthritis. IMAGE: Journal of Nursing Scholarship, Vol. 21(3), pp. 128-131.

Lorig, K.; Konkol, L., & Gonzales, V. (1987). Arthritis patient education: a review of the literature. Patient Education and Counseling, Vol. 10, pp. 207-252.

Manne, S.L. & Zautra, A.J. (1989). Spouse criticism and support: their association with coping and psychological adjustment among women with arthritis. Journal of Personality and Social Psychology, Vol. 56(4), pp. 608-617.

Montague, J. & Stein, V.R. (1989). Managing chronic pain. Dimensions in Health Services, Vol. 66(3), pp. 23-26.

Scott, D.L.; Symmons, D.P.; Coulton, B.L., & Popert, A.J. (1987). Long-term outcomes of treating rheumatoid arthritis: results after 20 years. Lancet, Vol. 1, pp. 1108-1111.

Seligman, M. (1975). Helplessness: on depression, development, and death. San Francisco. CA: W.H. Freeman.

The Older Woman with Diabetes Mellitus

Diana W. Guthrie, PhD, FAAN, CDE

SUMMARY. The human body wears out fast enough without the addition of a disease like diabetes that mimics a rapid, internal aging process. The older woman with diabetes faces multiple challenges, both physical and psychological. To control this life-threatening illness, she often is asked to participate in multiple self-care activities at a time when she needs or desires to slow down or do less–especially if a loved one has died. Or perhaps the care is given by nursing home personnel or family members. The health care professional working with her can be instrumental in helping her, or others involved in her care, to attain an improved quality of life. A good life in later years is possible for the diabetic woman, especially if small problems in self-care are addressed daily and thereby more complicated problems are prevented.

INTRODUCTION

Diabetes mellitus is no respecter of people, affecting young and old alike. It can be a very harsh disease or just an annoying one, depending in large part on the patient's self-care–taking medications faithfully, timing and distributing foods, and monitoring the body's responses through blood glucose readings and ketone testing. The expectation is a quality of life in the years when the body,

Diana W. Guthrie is affiliated with the University of Kansas School of Medicine-Wichita, 1010 N. Kansas, Wichita, KS 67213.

[Haworth co-indexing entry note]: "The Older Woman with Diabetes Mellitus." Guthrie, Diana W. Co-published simultaneously in the *Journal of Women & Aging* (The Haworth Press, Inc.) Vol. 5, No. 3/4, 1993, pp. 83-100; and: *Women and Healthy Aging: Living Productively in Spite of It All* (ed: J. Dianne Garner, and Alice A. Young), The Haworth Press, Inc., 1993, pp. 83-100. Multiple copies of this article/chapter may be purchased from The Haworth Document Delivery Center [1-800-3-HAWORTH; 9:00 a.m.-5:00 p.m. (EST)].

mind, and spirit may be battered by aches and pains rather than enriched by age and experiences.

Definition

Diabetes mellitus was first described as a "melting of the flesh." The disease has been with us since the earliest years of recorded history. Its name is very descriptive: diabetes–"to siphon through" and mellitus–"sweet tasting" (Bliss, 1982).

"Sugar" diabetes is considered a syndrome due to the multiple causes of the diseases. Type I, insulin-dependent diabetes, is considered an immunological disease occurring in a genetically susceptible person. Type II, non-insulin-dependent diabetes, is considered a genetic disease with an environmental association (Ratner, 1992).

Diabetes is believed to be due to a lack of relative availability of insulin, which aids in the metabolism of carbohydrates, proteins and fats. Inside the cell, insulin stimulates a glucose transportation protein. This triggers the biochemical mechanism within the cell that allows the glucose transportation hormone (GLUT) to proceed to the cell surface, where it biomechanically creates an opening large enough to permit glucose molecules to enter the cell (Garvey, 1992). Insulin also acts in a similar way to allow amino acids into the cell for protein synthesis. If glucose and insulin interact appropriately, fats are not mobilized as an alternate source of energy.

In many cases, for Type I diabetes, an autoimmune response leads to the initial triggering of the physiological process of diabetes. For Type II diabetes, the hyperglycemic state can lead to glucose toxicity in the beta cells and may kill them. The number of receptor sites, particularly on muscle cells, can decrease in number, as a protective mechanism against the presence of too much insulin. Insulin resistance through problems associated with the cell receptor sites and a down-regulation (or decreased number) of receptor sites could occur.

Another factor that may contribute to diabetes, independently or concurrently, is an increase in glucose production in the liver, which challenges the rest of the body to compensate. Diabetes can also result from the surgical removal of the pancreas or from the stress on insulin production caused by interaction with other diseases (such as cystic fibrosis or acromegaly), or medications (such as steroids). If the pancreas becomes fibrotic, perhaps from a long history of poor nutrition and/or alcoholism, a woman can also develop diabetes.

EPIDEMIOLOGY

Diabetes, especially Type II, is very common in the elderly. As people age, the incidence of diabetes increases with women having a higher prevalence (and incidence) than men.

In the general population, one in 20 people has diabetes. Among the elderly (those age 65 and over), 2 in 5 or 40% have diabetes (ADA, 1991). Under age 65, African-Americans have twice the incidence of diabetes and Hispanics three times the incidence as Caucasians. From age 65 on, the prevalence is much closer (Harris, 1987) (see Table I). The majority of people with diabetes in the United States have Type II diabetes (85-90%), with the remainder having Type I (10-15%). Most of those who have Type II diabetes are also overweight (approximately 85%-90%).

Risk Factors

Multiple risk factors are associated with diabetes. Obesity is the most obvious, but hypertension is often a close second. Smoking and chronic alcohol intake are also problems. Other risk factors are high cholesterol and triglyceride levels, inactivity, increased stressors, and any other physiological changes.

Symptoms

When a woman is older, diabetes may be less easily recognized. Frequent urination (polyuria) may be thought of as "a weak bladder," or "just another infection." Frequent drinking (polydipsia)

Table I

Age	Prevalence % vs sex and age 55-74					
	Black		Caucasian		Hispanic	
	M	W	M	W	M	W
55-64	14	25	9	15	28	31
65-74	29	23	18	16	24	40

may not be noticed if it occurs during the hot time of the year. Excessive eating (polyphagia) may be noted as "emotional eating" or just part of aging. A woman who has decompensated into Type I diabetes or is just developing the disease may react with joy to the symptoms: "I'm eating all I want and I'm even losing weight!"

Tiredness is usually the first symptom that prompts a woman to make a doctor's appointment. Elevated blood glucose levels can make her irritable, depressed, and tired. Pain in her extremities (neuropathy) is another reason a woman might seek help. Yet often diabetes is diagnosed when the older woman goes to the doctor for another reason. Dry skin and wounds that are slow to heal can be indications of diabetes. These symptoms of diabetes can be misinterpreted. Blurred vision, for example, might be attributed to aging. Yet cataracts develop 1.4 times more frequently in people who have diabetes. Bloating, aches and pains associated with aging, problems passing urine, and sexual dysfunction, could be symptoms of neuropathy.

DIAGNOSIS

The diagnostic norms were set, in the 1980s, at a higher level to keep from over-diagnosing individuals and to take into account the higher diagnostic criteria considered acceptable in older adults. The following table (see Table II) includes these diagnostic criteria.

An occasional blood sugar reading over 200 calls for a glucose tolerance test; 75g is the glucose load administered for the oral challenge after the fasting blood sugar has been obtained. A 115 or higher fasting should be looked on with suspicion even though the numbers noted in Table III are considered 2 standard deviations

Table II

Clinical Classifications for Diabetes		
Type of Diabetes	Initial Blood Glucose	Subsequent Tests
Type I Diabetes	Fasting >140 mg/dl	2 or more 200 mg/dl+
Type II Diabetes	Fasting >140 mg/dl	1 - 200 mg/dl+
	Fasting <140 mg/dl	2 or more 200 mg/dl+
Impaired Glucose	Fasting <140 mg/dl	1 - 200 mg/dl+
Suspicious	Fasting >115 mg/dl	1 hour >195 mg/dl
		2 hour >165 mg/dl
		3 hour >145 mg/dl

about the norm. In general, glucose intolerance is an expected possibility as a person ages, although age has not been officially noted as part of the detection process.

Testing for glucose in the urine, for diagnosis or for monitoring change, is of little value, especially in the older woman. The level at which glucose is "spilled" into the urine (renal threshold) increases as a person ages (normal threshold expectation is 160-180 mg/dl–a sixty-two-year old female did not demonstrate glucose in the urine until her blood glucose levels were well over 250 mg/dl). So, a person could have a negative urine test but have a blood glucose level of 300 mg/dl or even higher. Ketones are seldom present in the urine of people with Type II diabetes. In fact, the disease is sometimes called "ketosis-resistant diabetes." Yet ketone testing is still important, especially during illness or when blood sugars are 250 or above as the person might be decompensating to a ketosis-prone state.

ACUTE COMPLICATIONS

Although, Type II diabetes is a less severe form of the disease, end-stage kidney disease, amputation, and blindness can occur with the incidence of complications related to small blood vessel disease (kidney, eye). (For example, end-stage kidney disease occurs in 1 out of 20 who have Type II diabetes vs. 1 out of 4 with Type I diabetes). These are some of the chronic complications, but the acute complications (such as diabetic ketoacidosis, hyperglycemic hyperosmolar non-ketotic syndrome, and hypoglycemia) and intermediate complications (such as illness, surgery, psychosocial problems, and menopause) may also occur, usually not as frequently.

Diabetic ketoacidosis. The acute complication of diabetic ketoacidosis may be suspected with elevated glucose levels and the pres-

Table III

Small amounts of oils and sweets
2-3 servings of milk or milk products
2-3 one-ounce servings of meat, fish, poultry, and nuts
2-4 servings of fruits - 3-5 servings of vegetables
2-4 servings of fruits/ 3-5 servings of vegetables
6-11 servings of grains, rice, pasta

ence of ketones in the urine. If the blood glucose levels are above 600-800, hyperglycemic hyperosmolar non-ketotic syndrome may be the diagnosis (this may occur in an older person with Type II diabetes that may or may not have been diagnosed and is related to a state of severe dehydration in a woman who is non-ketosis prone).

Diabetic ketoacidosis might happen to a person who has decompensated from Type II into Type I diabetes or perhaps has Type I diabetes and is ill and is not taking enough insulin or oral hypoglycemic agent. Not only are the blood glucose and ketone levels elevated, but CO^2 and sodium are low, and serum potassium is low, normal or high. Dehydration is present and the rest of the electrolytes are imbalanced. The pH is depressed. Treatment is supported with insulin, fluids and electrolyte replacement.

Diabetes ketosis, a less severe state of this acidotic state, doesn't involve much of an imbalance of electrolytes; rather the hyperglycemia only sets the stage for further imbalance. Hyperglycemia and the counter-regulatory response (involving the secretion of epinephrine, norepinephrine, cortisol, growth hormone, thyroid-stimulating hormone, glucagon [and insulin in the person who does not have diabetes]) can be devastating to an elderly person. Epinephrine will increase blood pressure. If blood vessels have been previously damaged, an elevated blood pressure could lead to a heart attack (myocardial infarction), retinal hemorrhage, seizure, or stroke: muscular weakness/partial paralysis (hemiparesis).

Hypoglycemia. Hypoglycemia, another acute complication, may occur as a side effect of taking insulin or an oral agent. In the older person, renal inactivity or shutdown results in the need for less insulin and for some oral agents so hypoglycemia could occur.

Hyperglycemic hyperosmolar non-ketotic syndrome. If there is not enough insulin to control blood sugar, the third acute complication could result–hyperglycemic hyperosmolar non-ketotic syndrome ("syndrome" because these extremely high blood glucose levels do not necessarily lead to coma). Hyperglycemic hyperosmolar non-ketotic syndrome is even more dangerous. Extreme dehydration in the presence of elevated blood glucose levels of 600-800 mg/dl or greater and profound hyperosmolarity would lead to a poor prognosis. The small amount of insulin secreted is enough to prevent ketogenesis. Therefore, these individuals are very sensitive to small amounts of insulin.

INTERMEDIATE COMPLICATIONS

Illness, surgery, psychosocial problems, menopause, and periodontal disease are considered the intermediate complications for the elderly.

Illness. If healing has already been slowed, elevated blood glucose levels will result in even slower healing. If the blood sugars are high, antibiotics will have an even harder time controlling infection. Keeping the blood sugars near normal as much as possible during illness will prevent diabetic ketoacidosis.

Surgery. Older women who are hyperglycemic will heal more slowly from surgical procedures. An older woman should be directed to achieve at least high normal blood glucose levels both before and after surgery. If she doesn't, the availability of white blood cells will be decreased, and fibrinogen will be increased.

Psychosocial problems. Any psychological problem–whether adjusting to the loss of a loved one or adjusting to the diagnosis of various health problems (including diabetes)–will lead to fluctuations in blood glucose levels. Just as with surgery and illness, blood glucose levels need to be controlled. Hyperglycemia and hormonal changes may lead to depression. Hyperglycemia will contribute toward the drying of the vaginal wall. Without adequate lubrication (such as might be found with the use of water-soluble Abolene cream), her sexual activity may diminish due to discomfort.

The second group of challenges faced may be social. Family support may be absent, weak, or sporadic. Care may be a problem even if the older woman is in a nursing home (Mooradian, 1992). Overprotection might occur by a concerned spouse or other family member. A woman with no family support may need directed assistance to identify a support system, such as the American Diabetes Association. Knowledge may be lacking or inappropriately used. The self-care regimen may lead to confusion. A woman might forget when to take her medication or how much to take at that time. She may have difficulty handling a syringe or a blood glucose monitoring device. There may be difficulty in having enough money to purchase supplies.

Education of the family and counseling and support of the woman with diabetes are essential at any time in a woman's life. If the woman has developed a complication and becomes less mobile in relation to a usually active life, there is even more importance in having professional support to assist the woman to adjust to such a change in lifestyle.

Menopause. A woman who has Type I diabetes and is or is not on a cycle of estrogen and progesterone and is still menstruating, may have or start a history of markedly elevated blood sugars at the start of her period (which requires increased amounts of medication: insulin) and then a sudden drop as the menses progresses. As menopause progresses, "Hot flashes" often occur. Hot flashes can lead to elevated blood sugars. Treatment with estrogen and/or Vitamin E lowers the incidence of these uncomfortable physiologic responses, but the estrogen, in higher doses, may counter the lowering of blood glucose levels. Progesterone has been found to have no effect on blood sugars. Some older women with diabetes will not be treated with estrogens until their physicians are convinced that the chance of cancer is less than the possibility of cardiovascular disease and that the impact on blood glucose levels may be controlled with increased diabetes medication. More recent findings have demonstrated that low doses of estrogen apparently do not have much adverse effect on blood glucose levels. In fact, some find that estrogen enhances blood glucose control (Johnson, 1992).

Peridontal disease. It's a vicious cycle: hyperglycemia leads to poor healing and unhealthy gums; unhealthy gums and teeth lead to hyperglycemia. Appropriate dental care and normalized blood glucose levels can interfere with this cycle. General dental hygiene—with brushing, flossing, and rinsing—will promote a longer and healthier dental life.

CHRONIC COMPLICATIONS

Chronic complications are usually grouped into four classes: retinopathy, nephropathy, macroangiopathy, and neuropathy. The Centers for Disease Control have expanded these four classifications into nine areas that include more than chronic complications: psychosocial adjustment, acute complications (both of which have already been addressed), pregnancy (which is not an issue in this age group), periodontal disease (previously noted), eye disease (retinopathy), kidney disease (nephropathy), cardiovascular disease, or nerve disease (neuropathy), and foot problems. These complications are affected directly or indirectly by alterations in large and small blood vessel pathology, much of which is due to hyperglycemia.

Eye disease. Retinopathy is based on damage to single-cell-walled blood vessels on the retina, which leads to the development of collateral circulation (neovascularization). Extensive formation of new retinal blood vessels can lead to blindness. Basement membrane thickening is associated with the weakening of single-celled-walled blood vessels throughout the body. This action leads to the weakening of the blood vessels in the eyes, kidneys, and heart. When these weakened walls burst, hemorrhage occurs. If the new blood vessels enter into the fovea of the eye, blindness occurs.

Kidney disease. In the early stages of kidney disease, the pelvis and tubules of the kidney may stretch, caused by exacerbations of acutely elevated blood glucose levels. This "stretching" is believed to be an irreversible process that is worsened by hypertension. In normal aging kidneys, creatinine clearance may increase and then decrease (1 ml/month). Blood vessel damage due to hyperglycemia and disease (i.e., hypertension et al.) would speed up this process. This decrease in the creatinine clearance rate may be a sign of diabetes kidney complications or nephropathy.

Nephropathy involves basement membrane thickening leading to leakage of protein and hemorrhage. It may be preceded by, or exist concurrently with, another kidney disease, glomerulopathy. End-stage kidney disease usually involves both, although earlier stages of the disease may not.

Cardiovascular disease. Heart disease involves both large and small blood vessels. Large blood vessel disease may be due to high-density vs. low-density lipoprotein problems that are non-diabetes related. However, hyperglycemia can also contribute by increasing "platelet stickiness" that results in larger areas of blockage, as cholesterol covers the platelet aggregation on the injured inner lumen of the blood vessel wall. Disease of the myocardium (cardiomyopathy) is associated more with the smaller blood vessels. Strokes are perhaps more common with large blood vessel problems, but mini-strokes could be caused by damage to small blood vessels.

Neuropathy. Nerve disease involves the polyol pathway (also called the sorbitol pathway), and can affect the cells of the body, as noted in the classic work by Winegrad (1976). Neuropathy also involves the sodium/potassium shunt. This process (shunting of sodium and potassium) results in an electrical message alteration.

The polyol pathway occurs when there is not enough insulin to drive the glucose through its usual glycolytic pathway. When this occurs, there appears to be an increase in aldosreductase, an enzyme that enhances the development of sorbitol. Sorbitol, in the presence of sorbitol dehydrogenase, changes to fructose–the "useable" form of glucose. Whether myoinostital (an ingredient necessary for normal cell functioning) is blocked by sorbitol or the fructose/sorbitol concentrations result in an osmotic gradient, the "insulation" of the nerve is "lost" and the woman experiences discomfort. A woman may feel pain, tingling, or numbness as the erratic signals are sent through the altered sodium and potassium in her nerves. If bilateral peripheral nerves are involved it is called distal polyneuropathy. If one group of nerves is affected there is focal neuropathy (mononeuropathy), or if nerves throughout the body are affected, autonomic neuropathy. A few examples of autonomic neuropathy are bloating or a feeling of fullness (gastroparesis), diabetic diarrhea, a neurogenic bladder, and sexual dysfunction. Older women may also have cramps in their legs when they walk (intermittent claudication) that may or may not be diabetes-related.

Foot problems. As peripheral vascular disease (PVD) increases and neurological function decreases, a woman might not notice that she is standing on a piece of glass or a tack. As PVD progresses further, gangrene could occur and, in its "wet" form, result in the need for an amputation. So women need thorough, and perhaps repeated, counseling on proper foot care. A daily foot examination becomes a must. Keeping the feet clean is a close second. A third is cutting the toenails in line with the top of the toes. Visits to the podiatrist become one of the best preventive measures possible for the elderly woman who may be unable to care for her own feet.

MEDICATION OPTIONS AND ISSUES

Although many older women are given a diabetes management program termed, "diet alone," most will eventually need some kind of diabetes medication. Oral agents and insulin are the two treatments available.

The first-generation medications are the short-acting tolbutamide (Orinase), the intermediate-acting acetohexamide (Dymelor) and tolazamide (Tolinase), and the long-acting chlorpropamide (Diabinese). Acetohexamide and chlorpropamide are potentially more harmful to the older person, due to the toxicity of their breakdown products in the liver and, on kidney "shut-down," could lead to prolonged hypoglycemia.

The second-generation sulfonylureas are called gliburide (Diabeta, Micronase, and Glynase) and glipizide (Glucotrol). These medications are available in less concentrated dosages, and have fewer side effects. Gliburides are excreted 50% to the kidney and 50% to the bile. Glypisides are excreted 90% to kidney and 10% to the bile. In divided doses, 20 mg is considered the top dose for Diabeta and Micronase, while 12 mg is the top dose for Glynase; and 40 mg for Glucotrol.

Older people usually have little difficulty accepting an oral agent. The drawback is that an oral agent is not a lifetime treatment–the average length of time a person is on an oral agent is 5 years. The absorption rates of short-acting (regular & Semi Lente), intermediate-acting (NPH and Lente) and long-acting insulin (Ultralente) can be influenced by where the injection is given and whether the kidneys are fully functioning.

Most women who have diabetes on insulin need two or more doses daily in order to obtain 24-hour blood glucose control. One dose given before bedtime has been found useful in lowering the fasting blood sugar, thus making oral agents given during the day more effective for a slightly longer period. Other older people, with a lesser ability to rid insulin from the body, or for other reasons, may do well with a split mix twice a day (often 2/3 before breakfast & 1/3 before supper) in a premixed form (70 units NPH to 30 units Regular or 50 units NPH to 50 units Regular).

A major issue for many older women is third party coverage for the costs involved in maintaining wellness: the costs of medication, the machinery and/or strips to monitor the blood glucose levels, and adequate education by a Certified Diabetes Educator for both the diabetic woman and her significant other. Medicaid will cover medication and some strips, while Medicare will cover them in some states but not in others. Medicare will not cover prescribed orthopedic shoes, frequently found necessary to maintain neurologically involved feet. Education may be covered if the program has completed the rigorous review of self-recognition by the American Diabetes Association (includes the use of certified diabetes educators).

The health professional can be invaluable in directing these women to possible sources of financial help. Older people may go without medicine for days or weeks if they have no recourse to groups like the local medical society, a church group, or a low-income clinic.

STRATEGIES FOR PRODUCTIVE AND HEALTHY AGING

For the older diabetic woman, as for the rest of us, a major goal for the later years is to maintain a high quality of life. For this, she needs normal blood glucose levels (albeit, high normal levels) and the ability to understand and balance food, activity, and medication. The question is often asked, "Why normalize blood glucose levels in the elderly?" The answer is the common observation that when a diabetic gets used to normal levels, she feels better. It does take her a few weeks to get used to normal levels, especially if she has had elevated levels for months or years. On the other hand, too tightly controlled blood glucose levels could lead to frequent mild to severe hypoglycemia. Which alternative is more dangerous to the elderly person–elevated blood glucose levels or frequent hypoglycemia? This is still being debated, but most authorities accept the "high side of normal" as the appropriate goal (Morley, 1992) but an overall average of blood glucose levels should be below 150 mg/dg.

Exercise. The older diabetic woman must exercise, as her ability and physical condition permit. Exercise will lead to decreased depression, an increased sense of well-being, and an increased pain threshold. The goal should be 20-30 minutes of aerobic activity every day or every other day.

But the older woman needs to start slowly. The older she is, the slower the progression and intensity should be. An 80-year old woman who started water exercise by doing five, three-way leg-kick repetitions (front/side/back) was sore the next day. It took a month to get her back in the pool. This second time, she started with one three-way repetition on each side. The result: by the end of the summer, she was up to 20 repetitions in each direction.

Walking is also a recommended activity, but if weight or disability do not permit it, aerobic exercise can be achieved by rhythmic arm swings.

Meal planning. Little normalization of blood glucose levels can be achieved without the appropriate distribution of foods and sound nutritional choices. For normal nutrition, the older woman may need to eat smaller amounts more frequently rather than just two or three meals a day. Basic eating guidelines should be followed: (1) normalize blood glucose levels; (2) maintain a healthy weight; (3) decrease intake of fat; (4) increase fiber intake; (5) decrease protein, but include some protein in the bedtime snack; (6) distribute food throughout the day; and (7) choose nutritious foods. If a woman's cultural eating habits have included fatty foods, it will be most difficult to alter them at this older age. Asking for a decrease in fat intake, sweets, and weight, and an increase in fiber might be more than she can tolerate. Changing to these habits calls for creativity. Only one change should be the focus for each week or month.

Each woman who has diabetes needs an individualized dietary program. Looking at her usual food intake and the times she eats is the place to start. Improving nutritional intake comes second. Some methods for tracking nutritional intake are: the constant carbohydrates system (i.e., the person keeps the amount of carbohydrate in the meal plan at a set number with the intake of fats or proteins following recognized nutritional guidelines); the exchange system, which portions meat, fat, fruit, bread, vegetables, milk into interchangeable units; and the point system, a simplified method of calorie counting where 75 calories equal one point. The woman with diabetes daily meal plan should be designed around the recommended nutritional pyramid (see Table III) in relation to basal energy expenditure and activity needs.

Getting cooperation depends on the woman's perception of the need for change and her willingness to do it. If she feels in control by making meal plan decisions, she will be more apt to follow them.

Monitoring. Monitoring puts the whole self-care program together. Self-monitoring of blood glucose (SMBG) gives the direction and support for her self-management decisions. A sense of participation and empowerment aids in making choices.

Blood sugar readings may be taken at four times: fasting and 1-2 hours post-meal or pre-meal and at bedtime. At least one profile (a blood sugar taken at each of the four times) should be a minimum for the person with Type II diabetes unless the person is ill or under undue stressors. Three profiles per week are recommended for person with Type I diabetes. Daily blood sugar profiles are the recommended minimum for the person on an insulin infusion pump. The more normalized blood glucose levels desired, the more consistently blood glucose tests should be completed (3-4 times or more a day). (A major problem has recently occurred in nursing homes. Regulations now require a costly certification process so many nursing homes are choosing not to perform SMBG on their residents.)

If SMBG is refused, post-prandial urine glucose testing would be an option (the diabetic should empty her bladder before the meal and obtain the first void one to two hours after the meal). Higher blood sugars after eating could lead to some urinary excretion of carbohydrates (glycosuria), even with an elevated renal threshold.

A renal threshold may be assessed by repeating multiple urine tests concurrent with blood glucose tests (i.e., pre meal blood sugar test and urine test followed by "concurrent" blood sugar and urine tests at one, two and three hour intervals after the meal). The test is read diagonally, not horizontally. For example, 160 mg/dl and negative for glucose pre-meal; 360 and negative 1 hour post-meal; 220 and 2% at the two-hour time; and 200 and 1% at the three-hour time. The renal threshold is about 200 (normal 160-180 mg/dl). A woman could do this herself or this could be done in the office or hospital by a professional.

As noted before, ketone testing should be completed, even for those with Type II diabetes, when the woman is ill or when her blood sugars are greater than 240 mg/dl.

Glycosylated hemoglobin tests (Hgb A1c or Hgb A1) or fructosamine tests (or a glysylated serum protein test) give a range of mean blood glucose levels for the former (2-3 months) to the latter (approximately 7-10 days). This information can be used by the health professional to educate the patient/client or to assist the physician in making management choices. Although this is an office procedure, it is a part of the total monitoring process.

Medication management. There are four major approaches to management: (1) the "sliding scale" in which a blood sugar of a certain level means that no insulin or just a certain amount is to be administered; (2) the "algorithm" when, on a baseline of two or more doses of insulin, supplements are based on blood sugars of 150 or higher (i.e., 1 unit of insulin administered for every 50 mg/dl of blood sugar 150 or higher) (Skyler, 1981); (3) the "pattern approach," using the last 24-hour profile to predict her needs for the next 24 hours, or, at home, making decisions based on blood glucose records over the last three to five days to predict what would be needed for the next three to five days. The advantage is that all changes in dosage are made before elevated blood sugar is identified, ensuring that the woman does not make changes based on a single high reading unless she is ill (Guthrie, 1990); and (4) the "glucograf method" in which the individual is so familiar with her body's responses to food and insulin that she alters each dose, depending on her body's responses in relation to the expected activities of the coming hours (Berstein, 1981).

Education. In order to have ideal blood sugar, the mind and spirit must be taken into account as well as the body. Education helps in decision-making and also in recognizing that emotions may become involved. (Emotional stressors can increase blood glucose levels, and raised blood glucose levels can affect emotional responses.) Yet despite all its benefits, education can also result in fear. Fear can come about when a woman's awareness of the disease is increased. For example, a diabetic's fear might focus on anything from the possibility of having hypoglycemia in the middle of a bridge game to developing a debilitating chronic complication. Fear may lead to a reactive formation, where she will take less rather than more care of herself. Or fear could lead to compulsions that thwart her goal of a quality life.

Psychosocial strategies. Personal management of day-to-day activities vary. The question for the older woman is, "How can I do such-and-such an activity in spite of having diabetes?" The health professional might ask, "How can I assist the elderly woman in achieving a level of diabetes control to prevent the symptoms of both hypo- and hyperglycemia?" Pre-planning is the key in both cases, and it's most effective when the diabetic actively participates. The following scenario illustrates the point:

> An older woman develops a chronic complication. Here is a vibrant, always in control, leader, who is now dependent on those around her. Bitterness could be the inevitable outcome, unless the woman is directed to refocus her attention to those areas in which she still has some input. Scheduling, planning for, and recognizing physical responses are still in her control; she also may remind herself that she still has the support of family and friends to attain the quality of life desired.

A woman who has diabetes who brings along a family member or friend to an education class has taken a major step. She recognizes the teamwork needed to develop a healthy lifestyle. By being willing to share her concerns with another, she has taken a step away from denial. Another benefit of having a partner in class is the chance to get a "second opinion" when, after class, she tries to remember what was said.

Perhaps one more thing should be addressed. A husband, feeling sorry for his wife who has a chronic illness, may baby or smother her. He may unintentionally destroy her dietary control by pleading, "Just a little bite won't hurt." In addition, he, or friend or another family member, may fear losing her. Others' poor understanding of diabetes could lead her to poor self-care, resulting in poorer blood glucose control. Self-management and support go hand-in-hand to form the basis of quality health care. Support groups provide added education and support for the woman who has the desire to take advantage of them. Having a chance to talk to someone else who has experienced some of the same problems leads to a sense of belonging. Identifying such support may have to come from outside the family. If a diabetic woman is less able or willing to care for herself, then these supportive issues should become a part of the lives of others involved in her care.

CONCLUSION

The older woman with diabetes faces a number of threats–to her health and her quality of life. As she learns to change what she can and recognize what can't change (an adaptation of the Serenity Prayer), then she is better able to make intelligent choices. Positive health changes can lead to a better quality of life.

NOTE

Accredited educational programs have been approved by the American Diabetes Association. This organization awards the designation Certified Diabetes Educator to those who have completed the accreditation program. For a listing of Certified Diabetes Educators in your area, contact the American Association of Diabetes Educators, Suite 1240, 444 N. Michigan Ave., Chicago, IL 60611-3901; 1 800 338 3633. For a listing of programs that have achieved Self-Recognition contact the American Diabetes Association, 1660 Duke St., Alexandria, VA 22313; 1 800 232 3472.

REFERENCES

Bernstein, R.K. (1981). *Diabetes: the glucograf method for normalizing blood sugar.* Los Angeles: Jeremy P. Tarcher, Inc.

Bliss, M. (1982). *The discovery of insulin.* Chicago: University of Chicago Press.

Diabetes 1991 Vital Statistics (1991). Alexandria, VA: American Diabetes Association.

Garvey, W.T. (1992). Glucose transport and NIDDM. *Diabetes Care, 15*(3), 396-417.

Guthrie, D.W., & Guthrie, R.A. (1990). Approach to management. *The Diabetes Educator, 15,* 401-406.

Harris, M.I. (1990). Epidemiology of diabetes mellitus among the elderly in the United States. In J. Froom (Ed.), Diabetes Mellitus in the Elderly. *Clinics in Geriatric Medicine, 6*(4), 703-720.

Johnson, J.V., & Brumsted, J.R. (1992). Estrogen replacement therapy. *Diabetes Self-Management, 3,* 42-44.

Mooradian, A.D. (1992). Caring for the elderly nursing home patient with diabetes: a complex challenge to clinicians. *Diabetes Spectrum, 5*(6), 318-322.

Morley, J.E. (1992). Managing diabetes in the elderly. *Clinical Focus,* Sept., 23-28.

Ratner, R.E. (1992). Overview of diabetes mellitus. In D. Haire-Joshu (Ed.), *Management of diabetes melligus: perspectives of care across the life span* (p. 8). St. Louis: Mosby Yearbook.

Skyler, J.S., Skyler, D.L., Seigler, D.E., & O'Sullivan, M.J. (1981). Algorithms for adjustment of insulin dosage by patients who monitor blood glucose. *Diabetes Care, 4*(2), 93-318.

Winegrad, A.I., & Greene, D.A. (1976). Diabetic polyneuropathy: the importance of insulin deficient hyperglycemia and alterations in myoinostitol metabolism in its pathogenesis. *New England Journal of Medicine, 295*(25), 1416-1421.

Heart Disease and Older Women

Lois M. Rimmer, PhD, RN

SUMMARY. Heart disease has traditionally been thought of as a man's disease. However, one in three older women develop heart disease, making it the leading cause of death in older women. Current treatment for heart disease is based largely on studies using males as subjects. Doctors are just now beginning to learn about differences in men and women who have heart disease. The focus of this discussion is heart disease as it relates specifically to women. Risk factors considered are smoking, high blood pressure, elevated blood lipids, diabetes mellitus, obesity, stress, family history and physical inactivity. Diagnosis, treatment options and strategies for living productively with heart disease are presented.

Attention has recently been focused in both the popular and professional literature on heart disease as it relates specifically to women. Heart disease continues to be the leading cause of death in the United States for both men and women, but the most recent data from the American Heart Association show that cardiovascular disease and strokes combined claim the lives of more women than men (American Heart Association, 1992). In addition, women who suffer heart attacks are twice as likely as men to die within the first few weeks and have a higher chance of having a second heart attack within four years. One in three women over the age of sixty-five has some form of cardiovascular disease. Black women have a higher

Lois M. Rimmer is affiliated with Washburn University, Topeka, KS.

[Haworth co-indexing entry note]: "Heart Disease and Older Women." Rimmer, Lois M. Co-published simultaneously in the *Journal of Women & Aging* (The Haworth Press, Inc.) Vol. 5, No. 3/4, 1993, pp. 101-117; and: *Women and Healthy Aging: Living Productively in Spite of It All* (ed: J. Dianne Garner, and Alice A. Young), The Haworth Press, Inc., 1993, pp. 101-117. Multiple copies of this article/chapter may be purchased from The Haworth Document Delivery Center [1-800-3-HAWORTH; 9:00 a.m.-5:00 p.m. (EST)].

101

mortality rate from coronary heart disease than white women (American Heart Association, 1989).

Pre-menopausal women are far less likely to suffer from cardiovascular disease than men, but after age fifty, women develop cardiovascular disease at an increasing rate, reaching parity with men during their sixties. Since American women can now expect to live twenty-five or thirty years past menopause, this puts them at high risk for cardiovascular disease in their later years (Wellness Letter, 1992).

Although the overall rates of death due to cardiovascular disease have been declining over the past ten years, the absolute number of deaths remains high because of the increasing proportion of older persons in the population, and a significant proportion of this group are older women. Shron and Friedman (1990) point out that until recently, most epidemiological studies and clinical trials on heart disease excluded the very old and seldom studied persons over sixty-five. Dr. Marianne Legato, a cardiologist and researcher who is on the faculty of the Columbia University College of Physicians and Surgeons, reports that nearly every major cardiac research study has focused on male patients as subjects. An exception is the Framingham Heart Study, which has followed subjects since 1948 and whose subjects included both men and women, many of whom are now quite elderly. The National Institutes of Health now requests that scientists include women in their studies or risk not being funded (Legato & Colman, 1991).

The medical community is just beginning to recognize that heart disease is a major killer of older women and that there are differences in diagnosis, treatment and prognosis which have yet to be adequately understood. Risk factors are also being examined to determine if they apply equally to men and women. A *Saturday Evening Post* article quoted a Professor of Cardiology at the University of Pennsylvania who is also the editor of the medical textbook, *Heart Disease in Women*, as follows: "Heart disease in men is very different from heart disease in women. And that's not even really common knowledge among cardiologists yet. I treat my female patients based on mostly male studies and tell them, 'we just don't know a lot' " (Rosenthal, 1990, p. 26).

This discussion will focus on what is known about heart disease and women, focusing specifically on coronary artery disease (CAD). General terms will be defined, followed by a discussion of risk factors, diagnosis and treatment options. Considerations of special significance to women will be presented along with strategies for reducing risk factors and improving older women's chances for a productive life should heart disease occur.

DEFINITIONS

- *Heart Disease* is a general term covering all ailments of the heart, from heart attacks to congenital defects.
- *Cardiovascular Disease* is a broad term referring to disorders of the heart and circulatory system ("cardio" means heart, "vascular" means blood vessels. This includes hypertension, atherosclerosis, stroke, rheumatic heart disease, and other disorders.
- *Coronary Artery Disease (CAD)* refers to conditions that cause narrowing of the coronary arteries (atherosclerosis) so that blood flow to the heart is reduced. This results in coronary heart disease (CHD), damage to heart muscle caused by insufficient blood supply from obstructed coronary arteries. Permanent damage to, or death of, heart muscle is called a heart attack *(Myocardial infarction, MI)*. An insufficient supply of blood to the brain can result in a stroke. (University of California, Berkeley, Wellness Letter, 1992, p. 4)

Heart disease is the leading cause of death for both men and women. However, there are differences in the anatomy and lifestyle of women that affect susceptibility to heart disease as well as the course of the illness. First, women tend to be smaller than men. Their hearts are smaller and their coronary arteries (those that supply blood to the heart) are smaller and narrower. It may take less placque to block coronary arteries in women. Also, studies suggest that womens' coronary arteries may contract more vigorously than mens' in response to the same stress. Women are older than men when they are at their highest risk for heart disease, which may partially explain the higher death rate and more serious complications that some women experience. Since older women are more likely to be widowed or living alone when heart disease strikes, they may not have adequate emotional support to assist them in coping with the disease (Legato & Colman, 1991).

RISK FACTORS

Cigarette Smoking

Cigarette smoking is one of the most serious risk factors for both men and women. Murdaugh (1986) reviewed several studies of younger women who experienced heart attacks and found that data consistently showed cigarette smoking to be a significant risk factor for coronary heart disease and sudden death in women. Data from the large Boston-based Nurses' Health Study, which involved 120,000 female nurses as subjects, implicated cigarette smoking in 50% of heart disease cases (Rosenthal, 1990). The use of oral contraceptives in a woman who smokes increases her risk for developing coronary heart disease by 30 to 40%. Women who are smokers reach menopause two to three years earlier than nonsmokers, which adds to their risk for developing heart disease. A disturbing trend is that twenty-seven percent of women currently smoke and studies show an increase in smoking among teenage girls (Legato & Colman, 1991). The number of men smoking in the United States has recently declined, but the number of women who smoke has not (National Womens' Health Report, 1993).

Hypertension

Hypertension or high blood pressure afflicts one in three American adults. As women age, they are more likely to develop hypertension than men. More than half of all women over fifty-five have elevated blood pressure and this increases to more than two thirds of all women over sixty-five (American Heart Association, 1992). It is estimated that only about half of the women who are hypertensive know of their disease and only eleven percent receive treatment (Eaker et al., 1992). Persons with an arterial blood pressure in excess of 160/90 mmHg have been shown to have a fivefold increase in heart disease compared to those whose blood pressure was 140/90 mmHg or less. When hypertension is untreated it can cause damage to the innermost lining of the blood vessels. This facilitates the development of atherosclerosis (Beare & Myers, 1990).

Elevated Blood Lipids

Elevated levels of lipids or fats in the blood are another significant risk factor for the development of atherosclerosis and thus for coronary artery disease. The principal lipids in the blood are cholesterol, triglycerides and phospholipids. Lipids are transported in the blood by substances called lipoproteins. About sixty percent of the body's cholesterol is carried by LDL (low density lipoprotein). High levels of LDL are thought to produce arterial deposits in the blood and are associated with an increased risk for coronary artery disease. HDL (high density lipoprotein) is thought to clear cholesterol from the system. High levels of HDL or a high ratio of HDL to LDL are associated with a decreased risk for heart disease.

Women tend to have higher HDL levels than men. Estrogen tends to raise HDL levels, leading to speculation that estrogen protects premenopausal women from developing heart disease. High total blood cholesterol levels, those above 200 mg/dl (200 milligrams per deciliter) increase the risk of coronary artery disease for both men and women, especially if the HDL level is below 35 mg/dl. An Israeli study showed that women could enjoy good health with any level of cholesterol and LDL as long as HDL made up twenty-three percent of the total. Findings from the Lipid Research Clinics Follow-Up Study showed that except for age, the level of HDL cholesterol was the single most accurate predictor of cardiac disease in women (Rosenthal, 1990).

Elevated triglyceride levels are implicated as risk factors for development of heart disease in both men and women. Legato and Colman (1991) report that women are at risk for coronary artery disease with triglyceride levels greater than 190 mg/dl, while men's triglyceride levels are a risk factor when they approach 400 mg/dl. Alcohol raises blood triglyceride levels. Smokers have triglyceride levels that are nine percent higher than nonsmokers.

Diabetes Mellitus

Persons with adult onset diabetes mellitus have a higher risk for developing cardiovascular disease. According to the American Heart Association (1992), more than eighty percent of people with diabetes mellitus die of some form of heart or blood vessel disease. There is also data that suggest that diabetes mellitus increases the risk of coronary artery disease threefold in women and puts them at the same risk as men of the same age (Beare & Myers, 1990).

Obesity

Persons who are more than thirty percent over their ideal body weight are at a higher risk for development of coronary artery disease, as well as for non-insulin dependent diabetes and hypertension. Overall obesity is not as important as the pattern of weight distribution. Midsection obesity is more dangerous than that which is concentrated on the hips and thighs (Legato & Colman, 1991). A waist-hip ratio greater than 1.0 for men and .08 for women point to increased risk for coronary artery disease. A woman's waist measurement should not be more than eighty percent of her hip measurement (American Heart Association, 1992). In other words, it's better to be shaped like a pear than an apple.

Stress

Much has been written over the years about Type A aggressive behavior in males. Data from the Framingham study showed that Type A behavior was predictive of an increased risk for heart disease in both men and women. A lesser known finding from the study, however, was an increased risk of heart disease among Type B, or passive women, married to overly demanding Type A men (Legato & Colman, 1991). In a recent front page story in the nationally circulated newspaper, *USA Today,* Dr. Edward Diethrich of the Arizona Heart Institute reported that women in low status jobs in which they have little control may experience greater stress than women in higher status jobs (Painter, 1993). Based on her clinical experience treating women patients, Dr. Legato believes that unrelenting stress plays a major role in the onset of heart disease. A chapter in her book, *The Female Heart*, supports her position (Legato & Colman, 1991).

Family History

Persons whose fathers have had a heart attack before age fifty-six or whose mothers had one before age sixty are at increased risk for coronary artery disease. This risk is present for both men and women (Legato & Colman, 1991).

Physical Inactivity

Physical inactivity can lead to development of other risk factors, such as weight gain and a decrease in HDL levels. While most studies that demonstrated beneficial effects of exercise on the heart have been done using men as subjects, a study conducted by the Cooper Institute for Aerobics Research in Dallas showed that high levels of physical fitness (as determined by treadmill tests) were associated with a low risk of heart disease in women under sixty-five (Wellness Letter, 1992). Increasing one's physical activity may also have a positive effect on stress reduction, as well as play a role in lowering blood pressure and increasing HDL levels. Women who engage in moderate exercise, such as briskly walking a half hour a day three times a week, can lower their risk for development of heart disease (Legato & Colman, 1991).

DIAGNOSIS OF CORONARY ARTERY DISEASE

Symptoms of coronary artery disease may first occur in the form of chest pain known as angina pectoris. This occurs when the heart muscle doesn't get its needed blood supply. If blood vessels become narrowed due to partial blockage by atherosclerotic placques, decreased amounts of blood flow through the coronary arteries. Blood carries needed oxygen to the heart muscle tissues. The heart's response to lack of oxygen is the symptom of chest pain, which often occurs upon exertion.

Anginal pain is usually felt behind the upper or middle portion of the breast bone and commonly radiates to the left shoulder and down the arm. Less commonly, it may radiate to the right shoulder, the neck or the jaw (Beare & Myers, 1990). Some persons experience lack of oxygen to the heart without pain. This is known as silent ischemia, which places them at risk for heart attack with no previous warning. The first indicator of coronary artery disease in women is likely to be angina. First heart attacks are more likely to be fatal for women than for men. Women also have an increased incidence of silent MI. This makes them more vulnerable to heart failure, stroke and death (Eaker et al., 1992).

There is considerable evidence building that physicians haven't been taking chest pain in women as seriously as they do in male patients. A study conducted recently at the Einstein College of Medicine found that cardiologists were three times more likely to diagnose a woman's chest pain as being "in her head" as they were a man's. Doctors were ten times more likely to refer male patients with coronary artery disease for further testing to determine if surgery was needed than female patients (Legato & Colman, 1991). There is also considerable anecdotal evidence in the current literature to suggest that women themselves don't take chest pain seriously, often dismissing it initially as indigestion or muscle strain. Consequently, they delay in seeking treatment in the early stages of the disease.

When a woman does consult a doctor for complaints of chest pain, there may be no abnormal findings on physical examination if she is not experiencing chest pain at the time of the exam. During an attack of angina, the patient may experience increased pulse rate, changes in blood pressure, abnormal heart rhythms, electrocardiogram (ECG) changes, sweating, pallor, and feelings of apprehension and weakness. The changes in the electrocardiogram during an attack of angina diagnose the presence of coronary artery disease. Patients may be tested for ECG changes while exercising on a treadmill. In this test, a patient walks or jogs while monitors measure the heart's electrical activity.

Other diagnostic tests include coronary angiography, in which contrast dye is injected into the coronary arteries and x-ray pictures called angiograms are taken. This test is described as the "gold standard" for diagnosis of heart disease. Radioisotope imaging can also be performed, in which thallium 210, a radioisotope, is injected into the bloodstream. The heart muscle takes up the thallium. A scanning machine provides images of the heart muscle. Regions of poor perfusion will show up as cold spots (areas of absent radioisotope intake). This non invasive test can be used for diagnosis as well as post operatively to assess patency of coronary artery bypass surgery grafts (Beare & Myers, 1990).

TREATMENT OF CORONARY ARTERY DISEASE

The goal of treatment of coronary artery disease is to relieve the acute episodes of angina and prevent further attacks. The physician will perform a complete physical examination and evaluate the severity of the disease process. Treatment may begin with the use of drugs that increase blood supply to the heart along with changes in lifestyle that reduce risk factors for continued progression of the disease. In severe cases of angina, procedures such as the use of an Intra-Aortic Balloon Pump or Percutaneous Transluminal Coronary Angioplasty can be used to improve blood supply to the heart. Another approach for severe cases is the surgical procedure CABG (Coronary Artery Bypass Graft). Neither the use of drugs nor the above mentioned procedures cure the underlying atherosclerosis, but are designed to improve blood flow to the heart muscle.

Women patients may have different patterns of responses than men to diagnostic tests. Noninvasive tests have lower predictive accuracy in women. For example, in the treadmill test, false positives for diagnosis of heart disease occur in only 8% of males, but in 67% of women. In the test using radioisotope imaging with thallium, the camera rays have to pass through breast tissue, which can create a shadow mimicking a blockage. Noninvasive diagnostic tests tend to be more reliable in older women, but many older women cannot exercise to adequate intensity. Older women who are obese, habitually sedentary or chronically ill may not be able to tolerate exercise. Physicians may need to proceed to coronary angiography earlier with some women patients (Eaker et al., 1991).

Recent studies show, however, that women undergo coronary angiography, angioplasty and bypass surgery less often than men.

Some data also suggest that women subjected to invasive or surgical therapy do worse than men. Women have four times the risk of men for dying during or immediately after bypass surgery. Following surgery, women often have continued chest pain. One explanation is that women's smaller coronary arteries are more difficult to manipulate surgically. Studies are needed to determine which women will benefit most from bypass surgery.

IF A HEART ATTACK OCCURS

The aim of treatment for coronary artery disease is to prevent the ultimate consequence of the disease process, myocardial infarction, from occurring. Complete lack of blood supply to an area of the heart leads to death of tissue in the area surrounding the blocked coronary artery. Thrombosis or clotting in an atherosclerotic coronary artery causes ninety percent of MIs. The severity and prognosis of the MI depends on many factors, including the size and location of the thrombosis and whether or not collateral circulation has developed (Beare & Myers, 1990). Myocardial Infarction remains the leading cause of death in the United States. More than forty-eight percent of the approximately five-hundred thousand heart attack deaths each year are women (American Heart Association, 1992).

Should a woman have any reason to believe she is experiencing a heart attack, it is very important to seek medical attention as soon as possible. Women should not try to drive themselves to the hospital, but should have a friend or relative go with them if possible. The sooner that a heart attack victim gets to a hospital emergency room, the better the chances are that early intervention may reduce the chance of serious complications that can arise. If a heart attack is in progress, the patient will most likely be admitted to a special unit called a coronary intensive care unit. In some cases, it may be determined that a patient can benefit from the balloon angioplasty procedure or may need the bypass operation.

According to Dr. Legato, many patients who have been admitted to a coronary intensive care unit for treatment following a heart attack will be ready to leave the unit within twenty-four to thirty-six hours, unless they develop complications which could prolong their stay. They will most likely complete their hospital stay on a unit in which their heart rhythm is constantly monitored. Here they begin the rehabilitation phase of their recovery. Patients may be surprised that they are encouraged to be out of bed and walking slowly around the unit as soon as they can tolerate this. An exercise program should be tailored to each person's ability and slowly increased.

During the recovery period from a heart attack, whether or not a woman has had a balloon procedure or a bypass operation, she will need both physical and emotional support. The period following discharge from the hospital is often a frightening one, since the constant care and reassurance of the hospital staff are suddenly withdrawn, as is the constant monitoring of the heart rhythm. Many people are fearful of having another heart attack and are timid about resuming normal activities after they return home. Dr. Legato recommends that women who live alone have someone come and stay with them for a week or two. Some hospitals offer cardiac rehabilitation programs that continue on an outpatient basis, in which the patient returns to the hospital each day to exercise under the supervision of trained personnel. They also interact with other patients who are recovering and receive emotional support during this time. Some areas have Mended Hearts support groups that patients can attend (Legato & Colman, 1991).

The recovery period may also involve making changes in one's lifestyle that contributed to the heart attack. Some, such as giving up smoking, or sticking to a reduced fat and calorie diet, may be more difficult to achieve than others. The good news is that the heart muscle does mend and it is possible for many patients to resume many activities engaged in prior to the heart attack. Many recovering heart patients are able to work up to enjoying sports activities, even more strenuous ones such as tennis. Sexual relations with a spouse can usually be resumed safely after a month or two. The recovery period may vary depending on the severity of the heart attack and the amount of damage to the heart muscle. For some people, the changes in lifestyle initiated after a heart attack may actually improve the quality of their life (Legato & Colman, 1991).

STRATEGIES FOR A PRODUCTIVE LIFESTYLE
IN OLDER WOMEN

At the present time, many of the strategies for controlling or preventing coronary artery disease are the same for both men and women. One problem is that many women are simply not aware of the risk heart disease poses for them as they get older. According to Trudie Bush, an Epidemiologist at Johns Hopkins School of Hygiene and Public Health (Rosenthal, 1990), women are far more concerned about developing breast cancer, yet many more post menopausal women die of heart disease than breast cancer. A recent study by a nurse researcher suggests that some women are not paying attention to cardiac risk factors. McKillip (1992) studied a group of working women in Northeast Kansas ranging in age from twenty to seventy years whose jobs were predominately clerical. She found that cardiac risk factors were high, especially for those most easily modified by lifestyle.

Advice given to women in a recent issue of the *University of California, Berkeley Wellness Letter* (1992) includes the following:

1. Be aware of your family history. If you have close relatives who have had heart attacks, you may be at high risk and should seek medical screening.
2. Reduce the amount of fat in your diet, especially cholesterol.
3. Maintain your weight at recommended levels for your height and build.
4. Do not smoke cigarettes. Stop smoking if you currently smoke.
5. Include regular aerobic exercise in your daily and weekly routines.
6. Have blood cholesterol and blood pressure levels checked at regular intervals.

There are some additional strategies which are currently under investigation. In men, taking aspirin daily has been shown to decrease the risk of a second heart attack. A study is currently in process which is investigating use of aspirin, beta carotene and Vitamin E in forty thousand nurse subjects to determine their relationship to prevention of heart disease (Allison, 1992). At present it isn't clear if taking one aspirin per day is as protective for women as for men.

The use of post menopausal estrogen therapy as a strategy for preventing heart disease in women is also being investigated. Thus far, evidence is inconclusive and it isn't known if the benefits outweigh the risks. A current study underway at the National Heart, Lung and Blood Institute, The Post Menopausal Estrogen/Progestin Intervention Trials, began in 1989 and should answer many of the questions, but results won't be available for several years (Legato & Colman, 1991).

Light to moderate use of alcoholic beverages may reduce the risk of heart disease. In a recent issue of *US News and World Report*, Dr. Charles Hennekens, an epidemiologist at the Harvard Medical School, stated that protective HDL cholesterol is markedly increased by alcohol. Persons who drink alcohol in moderate amounts have a lower risk for heart disease than non drinkers. He doesn't recommend that non drinkers start drinking, but persons who currently drink one or two drinks per day don't need to stop. Heavy drinkers, however, have a higher risk for heart disease (*US News and World Report*, October 5, 1992, Special Supplement).

LIVING PRODUCTIVELY WITH HEART DISEASE

Experiencing a heart attack or being diagnosed with coronary artery disease does not mean the end of satisfying and productive lifestyles for women. Treatments are available and adjustments can be made which control the progression of the disease. Many older women live active and enjoyable lives with a diagnosis of coronary artery disease. A woman's attitude toward making needed adjustments and working with her physician to find the best treatment plan for her are both very important.

Should a woman experience anginal pain, her treatment plan would most likely include medication to control the pain. A drug that is frequently prescribed to be taken at the onset of an anginal attack is oral nitroglycerine. When placed under the tongue, this drug quickly dilates arteries, allowing more blood to flow through the heart. Patients are advised to carry this medication with them at all times. If the anginal pain is chronic, a skin patch which slowly releases the drug over a twenty-four hour period can be worn. Women usually become aware of which activities or emotionally charged situations are most likely to trigger an angina attack, in which case they may take a nitroglycerine tablet beforehand to prevent an attack from occurring.

Other drugs are also available, such as beta blockers which block the effect of the sympathetic nervous system on the heart muscle or calcium channel blockers, which reduce the flow of calcium to the muscle cells in the walls of the coronary arteries, reducing spasms that cause anginal pain. Angina can often be treated successfully with medication and common sense strategies such as getting enough rest, minimizing stressful situations when possible and being aware of early warning signs that an attack may be impending. The doctor needs to be notified if changes in the pattern of the angina occur, such as increases in frequency or intensity of the pain (Legato & Colman, 1991).

Exercise is an important component of living productively with coronary artery disease. Exercise improves the tone of remaining heart muscle in persons who have suffered a heart attack, and can have beneficial effects in slowing progression of coronary artery disease. Exercise also helps build self esteem. The emotional effect of being diagnosed with coronary artery disease or having suffered a heart attack may lead to depression and despair about the quality of life that can be expected in the future. Participation in an exercise program often has the effect of turning around this downward emotional tailspin. Dr. Legato states, "Ironically, many women actually feel much better about themselves during the post-heart attack period than they ever did before (Legato & Colman, 1991, p. 206). Women should consult with their physicians about the type and intensity of exercise that is right for them.

Sometimes the emotional effects of suffering a heart attack or being diagnosed as having coronary artery disease are overwhelming at first. If there are unusually severe stresses in a woman's life or a very strong and sustained emotional reaction, a referral for short term psychotherapy may be helpful. Her family's response may have an effect on a woman's emotional state. For example, if her family becomes very overprotective, it may have a negative impact on a woman's emotional response to her illness. Some people initially respond to a heart attack by becoming extremely fearful that they will have another heart attack, causing them to become what is known as a "cardiac cripple." Keeping open lines of communication with her physician and participating in a support group may be very helpful in restoring confidence in her ability to recover and resume former activities.

Women who have been caregivers all during their lives may have difficulty accepting support or help from others. A strategy that Dr. Legato uses with her patients is to have them compose a wish list of everything in life they want just for themselves. Many women have difficulty in starting, but once over the initial roadblocks, find that this exercise has a very positive effect on the way they view themselves. Dr. Legato believes that learning to care about herself is an important first step for a woman in learning to take better care of herself (Legato & Colman, 1991).

Learning to live with coronary artery disease often includes making some dietary changes. This may be very difficult to accomplish since food patterns have usually developed slowly over many years. Women who cook meals for their families that are high in fats, calories and salt may be reluctant to change the family's eating patterns to accommodate their needs. Not only do women need to change their diets to reduce cholesterol and triglyceride levels, but they often need to reduce overall calorie intake to facilitate weight loss. In starting a program to change dietary habits, a helpful strategy is to keep a diary of all foods and beverages consumed for a week. Looking at one's own pattern of foods eaten helps to pinpoint areas that need changing. It may not be advisable to make drastic changes all at once, but rather to start with two or three areas and make small changes and then if those are successful, gradually add others. Sometimes, small dietary changes combined with increased exercise can produce beneficial results that are very encouraging (Legato & Colman, 1991).

Whatever strategies a woman uses to manage her coronary artery disease, maintaining open communication with her physician is very important. Many older women tend to be intimidated or fearful in the presence of a physician, so it is important to choose a physician that she feels comfortable with in discussing her symptoms. Financial considerations may also be a deterrent for older women with limited resources. They may be reluctant to schedule visits to the doctor unless a crisis occurs, or not take prescribed medications because of their high cost. This can be detrimental to successful management of their disease. Women with coronary artery disease who are reluctant to talk with their own physicians can use Dr. Legato's book, *The Female Heart*, as a good source of information. All aspects of coronary heart disease are covered in great detail in language that lay persons can readily understand. Reading this book could have the effect of giving a woman the confidence to know what questions she should be asking her own physician. The more informed a woman is about heart disease, the better able she will be to take an active part in the management of her disease.

It seems clear that questions relating to older women and heart disease are being increasingly addressed in scientific studies. The popular press is getting the word out to the general public about the risk heart disease poses for women. In the next ten years, data from studies currently in progress should shed new insights on the similarities and differences of Coronary Artery Disease in women and men, providing clearer guidelines for women for both prevention and treatment of this major health threat in their later years. In the meantime, women can help themselves by paying attention to the risk factors and modifying their lifestyles to minimize their risks for heart disease. Those women who develop coronary artery disease can become informed about their disease process and actively pursue strategies to maintain and improve their quality of life.

REFERENCES

Allison, M. (1992, April). Cardiovascular disease: A woman's heart. *Harvard Health Letter, 17*(6), 5-7.

American Heart Association. (1989). *Silent epidemic: The truth about women and heart disease*. Dallas: American Heart Association.

American Heart Association. (1992). *Heart and stroke facts*. Dallas: American Heart Association.

Beare, P. & Myers, J. (1990). *Principles and practice of adult health nursing*. St. Louis: CV Mosby Co.

Eaker, E., Johnson, W.D., Loop, F. & Wenger, N. (1992, February 15). Heart disease in women: How different? *Patient Care, 26*(3), 191-204.

Interview: Women, men and heart disease. (1992, October 5). *US News and World Report*, Special advertising section, total health.

Legato, M.J. & Colman, C. (1991). *The female heart.* New York: Simon & Schuster.

Long, P. (1991, March-April). A woman's heart. *In Health,* p. 53- 56.

McKillip, P.L. (1992). *Assessment of women's cardiac risk factors and the relationship of lifestyle habits for development of health promotion education.* Unpublished doctoral dissertation, Kansas State University, Manhattan, KS.

Painter, K. (1993, February 10). Heart disease: women's hidden threat. *USA Today,* pp. 1A, 2A, 4D.

Rosenthal, E. (1990, January-February). Heart disease: Women at risk. *Saturday Evening Post,* pp. 26-30.

Schron, E.B. et al. (1990). Cardiovascular options for the 90's. *Geriatric Nursing, 11*(4), 187-190.

Women and cardiovascular disease. (1993, January-February). *National Women's health report, 15*(1), 1-10.

Women and heart disease. (1992, February). *University of California Berkeley Wellness Letter,* pp. 4-5.

Women, Aging, and Cancer

Janet E. Lord, PhD, RN
Chris Richards, RN, MSN, OCN

SUMMARY. Women over 65 bear high risk for developing cancer. The risk for developing most cancers grows with increasing age. Of the 1.13 million people estimated to develop cancer in 1992, 362,000 (32 percent) will be women over 65 years old (American Cancer Society, 1992). The few early detection and prevention programs that have focused on this age group have found that the women often have problems with utilization, misconceptions, and plain lack of correct information. Treatment for women over 65 with cancer may differ from that for younger women because of age bias, comorbidity, stage of disease at time of diagnosis, and a lack of research on women of this age. Even quality of life and survivorship for the woman over 65 become issues due to the lack of knowledge about how women over 65 view these concepts. The Healthy People 2000 Report has developed goals for a healthier society by the year 2000. The priority areas in relation to cancer include reduction in cigarette smoking, dietary changes, greater utilization of early detection mechanisms, and decreasing exposure to occupational and environmental carcinogens. Implementation of these goals should affect future generations in terms of healthy aging: however, specific programs do need to focus on the woman over 65 and her present needs which will impact current and future health status.

The word cancer can stimulate a multitude of emotional responses from fear and dread to denial and sadness. Almost every woman has

---

Janet E. Lord is Associate Professor and Chris Richards is Clinical Instructor at the University of Arkansas for Medical Sciences, College of Nursing, Little Rock, AR.

[Haworth co-indexing entry note]: "Women, Aging, and Cancer." Lord, Janet E., and Chris Richards. Co-published simultaneously in the *Journal of Women & Aging* (The Haworth Press, Inc.) Vol. 5, No. 3/4, 1993, pp. 119-137; and: *Women and Healthy Aging: Living Productively in Spite of It All* (ed: J. Dianne Garner, and Alice A. Young), The Haworth Press, Inc., 1993, pp. 119-137. Multiple copies of this article/chapter may be purchased from The Haworth Document Delivery Center [1-800-3-HAWORTH; 9:00 a.m.-5:00 p.m. (EST)].

119

been touched by the loss of a loved one from cancer or lives with the fear of a recurrence of cancer in herself or a loved one. Currently one in three persons will suffer from cancer in their lifetime (American Cancer Society, 1992). Women are at risk for developing cancer of the lung, colon or rectum, breast, cervix and uterus, as well as others. As people age their risk for developing most kinds of cancers increases (American Cancer Society, 1992). This overview of cancer and older women explores the risk for lung, colorectal, breast, cervical, and uterine cancer as well as prevention and early detection, screening issues, treatment and survivorship, and goals for the 21st century.

BACKGROUND

Demographics show that 12 percent (24 million) of the population in the United States is over 65 with an approximate life expectancy of 75 (McCaffrey Boyle et al., 1992). Women comprise the majority of the over sixty-five population with one third of them living alone. While making up 12 percent of the population, the over 65 population has 57 percent of all the cancer (Ries et al., 1991). In 1992, 1.13 million people were projected to develop cancer. With 57 percent of these occurring in persons over 65, and the majority of persons over 65 being women, the risk of cancer in aging women is obviously high. The 1992 estimates for new cases of cancer for specific sites and total cases appear in Table 1 (American Cancer Society, 1992).

RISK FACTORS, PREVENTION, AND EARLY DETECTION

A causal relationship exists between cigarette smoking and lung cancer. Women who smoke are much more likely to die of lung cancer than women who do not smoke. A study of 619,225 women from 1982-1986 revealed that the women smokers were 12.7 times more likely to die of lung cancer than nonsmokers. This figure rose to 17.6 times if the woman also had a history of chronic diseases

TABLE 1

Estimated New Cancer Cases for Women, 1992

AGE	Lung	Colon	Breast	Cervical	Uterine	ALL Cancer Sites
65-69	12,000	7,100	23,800	1,000	6,800	91,000
70-74	12,000	8,700	22,000	900	6,000	98,000
75-79	8,300	9,800	19,300	700	4,300	83,000
80-84	5,000	9,000	12,700	500	2,600	53,000
85+	3,000	9,600	10,800	500	2,000	37,000
TOTAL	40,300	44,200	88,600	3,600	21,700	362,000

and rose to 22.0 times if the woman smoked 31 or more cigarettes per day (Garfinkel & Stellman, 1988). Seventy-nine percent of lung cancers in women are associated with smoking and, therefore preventable (American Cancer Society, 1992). When a woman stops smoking, her cancer risk drops to nearly the same point as a non-smoker. This finding holds true for women over 65 as well (Pathak, Samak, Humble & Skipper, 1986).

Lung cancer represents one of few cancers that has a known cause and is preventable. Early detection, on the other hand, is not state of the art. There are not good early detection screening methods, and by the time a person is symptomatic, the cancer is usually well advanced. On a slightly more positive note, smoking in women is on the decline from 32 percent in 1976 to 27 percent in 1987 (American Cancer Society, 1992).

The cause of colorectal cancer remains unknown. Risk factors include age, personal or family history of cancer, polyps of the colon or rectum, and inflammatory bowel disease. High-fat and/or low-fiber diet are other suspected risk factors (American Cancer Society, 1992).

The early detection/screening methods available for colorectal cancers consist of digital rectal examination, proctosigmoidoscopy, and stool blood test. The digital rectal examination will pick up approximately one-third of rectal and distal colon tumors; examination of the colon with a lighted scope (sigmoidoscopy) will reveal 50 percent of tumors (Luckmann & Sorensen, 1987); and the predictive value of stool blood test increases with age with a positive test indicating a 60 percent risk in older age groups (Winawer, Schottenfeld & Sherlock, 1988). However, use of stool blood testing in screening programs has some flaws. According to Simon (1985), the sensitivity and specificity of the test is relatively low, which means that tumors are overlooked (false-negatives) and too many people have to undergo unnecessary colon examinations because of false positives.

Again, with breast cancer no known cause exists. Major risk factors include age, country of birth, and history of breast cancer in both a mother and a sister. All other risk factors for breast cancer reported to date have a relatively modest impact (Kelsey & Gammon, 1991).

For early detection, recommendations are that women over 65 do monthly breast self-examination (BSE), have annual mammograms, and physical examinations (American Cancer Society, 1992). The American Geriatric Society recommends mammograms every two to three years for women age 65-85 (Clinical Practice Committee: American Geriatrics Society, 1989).

While cervical cancer is not a major cause of cancer illness or death in women over 65 (approximately 3,500 new cases and 2,500 deaths in 1990), the deaths are largely preventable and therefore an issue when discussing cancer and women over 65 (Blesch & Prohaska, 1991). Additionally, 41 percent of all cervical cancer deaths occur in women over 65. Risk factors include starting intercourse at an early age, multiple sex partners, and certain sexually transmitted diseases. For cancer of the uterus, history of infertility, failure to ovulate, prolonged estrogen therapy, and obesity are risk factors.

Early detection of cervical cancer involves a pelvic examination with the highly effective Papanicolaou smear test (Pap smear). ACS recommends that women over 18 have an annual pap test and pelvic examination and after three or more consecutive normal findings at the discretion of the physician (Mettlin & Dodd, 1991). The American Geriatrics Society recommends a pap test every three years until the age of 70 and notes that beyond 70 there is little evidence to suggest any benefits from continued pap tests (Clinical Practice Committee: American Geriatrics Society, 1989). Women at high risk for uterine cancer should have endometrial tissue sample examinations (American Cancer Society, 1992).

CANCER SCREENING AND WOMEN OVER 65

The statistics quoted previously about 57 percent of cancer occurring in the over 65 population and additionally, 60 percent of the deaths (Yancik, Kessler & Yates, 1988), indicate the need for cancer prevention and early detection programs for older women. However, according to Yancik, Kessler, and Yates (1988) health care providers have not shown a great interest in providing prevention and early detection programs for the elderly. Additionally, Rimer et al. (1983) found that the over 65 population "hold a number of beliefs and negative attitudes that might keep them from seeking treatment for potential cancer symptoms" (p. 384). The investigators further noted that cancer prevention and early detection programs often do not match the educational, physical, and lifestyle needs of persons over 65.

Of the three methods available for early detection of colorectal cancer, the most convenient and least expensive is the fecal occult blood screen (testing the stool for hidden blood). The Centers for Disease Control (1987) reports that of persons over 40, 25 percent of African-Americans and 15 percent of European-Americans had never heard of the test and that only 39 percent had ever had the test. Reasons given for avoiding the test include the unpleasant nature of feces and lack of understanding about its value (Box et al. in Weinrich, 1990). Weinrich (1990) found that the main predictor for using and returning the fecal occult test was gender. Women were much more likely than men to return the samples. Besides gender, the ability to use the telephone, shop for groceries or clothes, and clean house also were associated with return of the tests.

Harris et al. (1991) surveyed 1163 women and found that few women (20%), regardless of age, knew that the risk of breast cancer increased with age, older women tended to worry less about breast cancer than younger women, older women were less likely to have heard of mammography, and older women were less likely to know that mammography was better than physical examination for early detection. From this survey of women in North Carolina, only 26 percent of women over 70 reported mammography use in the past year compared with 32 percent of women in their 60s.

Researchers have also explored the use of cervical screening by women over 65. Celentano (1989) reports from a telephone survey of Maryland women that 19.3 percent of women over 65 had never had a pap test, with an additional 9 percent not having one for greater than ten years and 10.6 percent not having one for 5-10 years. Multifaceted reasons account for these results according to Celentano: recommendations for frequency of tests for women over 65 have changed 3 times in the last 10 years; women over 65 do not use obstetrician/gynecologists, the group of specialists most likely to do gynecologic screening; women do not avail themselves of screening; and physical constraints, such as arthritis, make a pelvic examination difficult for some women and their physician.

TREATMENT

It is beyond the scope of this text to provide an extensive review of all treatment regimens utilized in cancer therapy; however, specific treatment options for lung, colorectal, breast, and gynecological cancers are provided.

Many factors influence the treatment plan of cancer patients. Age and stage of disease are two of those factors. Though there is not a lot of information available on the relationship between age, stage of disease and choice of treatment for the older women with cancer, there is increasing evidence that older adults do not receive the same care as younger patients. This bias focuses on treating the patient based on their chronological age rather than physiologic age (Greenfield, Aronow, Ganz & Elashoff, 1989).

For the older woman with lung cancer, her presentation, degree of symptoms at the time of diagnosis, and the particular cell type of lung cancer determine her treatment. Because 90 percent of primary lung tumors originate from the bronchial epithelium, these cancers are collectively termed bronchogenic carcinomas. Lung cancer falls into two broad categories, small cell and nonsmall cell carcinomas. Each of these cell types takes a distinctly different natural course, and requires a separate approach for treatment. Oncologists assume the presence of metastatic disease in the fast growing small cell carcinoma at the time of diagnosis, even without objective evidence of disease spread. Hence, treatment of small cell carcinoma involves systemic therapy with combination chemotherapy. Nonsmall cell tumors grow slower and metastasize later; as a result, treatment depends upon the stage or extent of the disease at the time of diagnosis (Elpern, 1987). For the earlier stages of nonsmall cell lung cancer, surgery is usually the treatment of choice; in the later stages, palliation is usually the goal and includes different modalities such as surgery, chemotherapy, and/or radiation (Elpern, 1987).

The primary modality of treatment used for colorectal cancer is surgical resection. Regardless of the anatomic location of the tumor, the surgeon attempts to not only eliminate the tumor, but also any routes of metastasis. The primary reason for failure of surgical resection alone in colon cancer is local or regional recurrences.

Researchers have proposed adjuvant therapy using both radiotherapy and chemotherapy. To date, better results have occurred with radiotherapy. Clinical trials have indicated that preoperative irradiation decreases the size of the tumor thus making previously unresectable lesions resectable. Clinical trials with a variety of chemotherapeutic drugs have yielded some positive results in individuals with advanced, yet resectable tumors or metastatic disease. The drug of choice is 5-Fluorouracil[R](5FU). Despite clinical trials administering this drug in varying dosages, varying stages of disease, and different routes, the overall response rate is only 15-20 percent (Boarini, 1987).

Despite the advances in breast cancer treatment, controversy remains regarding the best type of therapy. When considering treatment options for breast cancer, the health care provider must include two factors: the modalities of treatment available and the stage of disease (Goodman, 1987). Possible methods of treatment include surgery, chemotherapy, radiotherapy, endocrine therapy, or some combination of these methods.

Cure is the goal of therapy for women diagnosed with local minimal disease and no evidence of metastasis. "The problem in breast cancer is not so much local control, but prevention of recurrence at distant sites" (Goodman, 1987, p. 450). The Modified Radical Mastectomy stands as the surgical treatment of choice for those women with more advanced, yet operable disease.

Because of the lack of cure associated with surgery alone, the incorporation of other treatment modalities becomes a necessity (Goodman, 1987). Most medical oncologists add chemotherapy to the treatment regimen of women with lymph node involvement, however, some controversy exists about whether postmenopausal women should receive chemotherapy even if they have lymph node involvement. Generally, pre- and perimenopausal women are more responsive to chemotherapy than postmenopausal women. This is most likely due to the fact that the disease in postmenopausal women is usually less aggressive than disease found in pre- and perimenopausal women. Another factor influencing the use of chemotherapy is whether or not the tumor is hormone receptor negative or positive (Goodman, 1987). The response rates for the use of single agent chemotherapy drugs is only between 20-30 percent, therefore, oncologists frequently employ a combination of drugs with a response rate of 50 percent (Goodman, 1987).

Because steroid hormones influence normal mammary tissue growth, the use of endocrine therapy stands as one of the major forms of treatment for women with metastatic breast cancer. Each normally-functioning mammary cell has receptor sites for each of the hormones that influence its growth and development. If the tumor cells are hormonally dependent, steroid hormones can actually promote the growth of breast cancer. For this reason, hormone receptor status is determined and is either estrogen receptor positive or negative (ER+/−), and progesterone receptor positive or negative (PR+/−). Tamoxifen (Nolvadex), an antiestrogen, currently is the first-line hormone therapy for postmenopausal women with metastatic disease and an ER+ tumor (Goodman, 1987). Radiation therapy, a local form of treatment, serves as a primary mode of therapy in early stages of breast cancer, as well as in conjunction with other modalities, in the treatment of more advanced disease (Goodman, 1987).

Is treatment for the older woman with breast cancer different than for younger women? Cases reviewed by Donegan (1983) indicated that treatment varied between older and younger women with breast cancer. It was anticipated that the older woman would present with more advanced disease, however, in this particular study, that was not the case. Clinical features in both the younger and older women were very similar. What did differ between the two groups was the higher frequency of other diseases in the older women. This issue of associated diseases (such as heart disease, hypertension, diabetes mellitus), known as comorbidity, appears to be an influential factor in choosing cancer treatment for the older woman. The use of adjuvant therapy following surgery declined with age, along with the use of systemic chemotherapy in women over the age of 65, even if documented axillary metastasis was present. Mastectomy is considered relatively low risk surgery, however in this study, postoperative mortality was found to be higher in the very elderly. As a result, less than optimal treatment was sometimes used in the older woman with breast cancer (Donegan, 1983).

Two types of gynecological cancers that women experience are cervical cancer, which usually occurs in women during their child-bearing years, and uterine endometrial cancer, which is considered a postmenopausal disease (Miller & Pazdur, 1987).

Following the diagnosis of invasive cervical cancer, the stage of the disease is established and the treatment plan is determined based on the women's general medical condition, age, extent of cancer, and presence of any complicating abnormalities. Each stage of the multi-stages of cervical cancer employs some form of hysterectomy in combination with radiotherapy unless the goal of therapy is strictly palliation, then the combination of treatments may not be used (Miller & Pazdur, 1987).

Factors influencing the treatment options for endometrial cancer include the stage of the tumor, the medical condition of the woman, the size of the uterus, and the histologic type and degree of differentiation of the tumor. Cornerstone therapy for endometrial cancer includes a total abdominal hysterectomy with a bilateral salpingo-oophorectomy with the possible addition of whole pelvis radiation and hormonal therapy for more advanced disease. Both single agent and combination chemotherapy regimen trials have produced varying responses (Miller & Pazdur, 1987).

STRATEGIES FOR PRODUCTIVE AND HEALTHY AGING

As one considers the many components of productive aging, key issues begin to surface when merging the ideas of productive living and cancer in the older woman. Issues such as survivorship and quality of life, reducing the risk of cancer, strategies for living with cancer, and the role of health care providers need to be addressed.

Survivorship and Quality of Life

In a medical community dominated by diagnosis and treatment of disease, the concepts of survivorship and quality of life are now emerging as important issues related to cancer care (Dow, 1990; Welch-McCaffrey, Hoffman, Leigh, Loescher & Meyskens, 1989; Quigley, 1989; Hoffman, 1989; Foreman & Kleinpell, 1990; Loescher, Clark, Atwood, Leigh & Lamb, 1990; Schmale et al., 1983).

Despite the increase in research and publications, a literature review revealed only one article (Foreman & Kleinpell, 1990) on the quality of life in older cancer patients, and no articles specifically on cancer, aging, women, and survivorship or quality of life. With this in mind, a general overview of survivorship and quality of life issues in the oncology population, with inference and application made to the aging woman with cancer as appropriate will be addressed.

In a broad sense, authors have described survival most often in the context of highly traumatic events that involve close touches with death, such as natural disasters or concentration camp experiences. Only in recent years have authors described survival to acute and chronic illnesses (Dow, 1990). The earliest discussion of long-term survival in oncology occurred in the pediatric literature, and was defined as a disease free state for five years after the time of diagnosis. This definition is not as clear cut in the adult literature (Quigley, 1989).

Quigley (1989) places the psychosocial consequences of cancer in two categories: emotional consequences and social consequences. While nothing indicates that severe psychopathology occurs with the cancer experience, evidence supports the occurrence of anxiety and depression (Dow, 1990; Welch-McCaffrey, Hoffman, Leigh & Loescher, 1989; Hoffman, 1989; Foreman & Kleinpell, 1990; Loescher, Clark, Atwood, Leigh & Lamb, 1990; Schmale et al., 1983). The person experiences a prevailing fear regarding the uncertainty of the disease free state–a nagging question about whether the cancer will return. Coupled with this uncertainty, the patient is preoccupied with physical complaints, especially fatigue and sexual dysfunction. Psychological distress or physiologic sequelae of the disease or treatment may trigger these symptoms. Many cancer survivors experience alterations in self-esteem and body image (Quigley, 1989).

Socially, the cancer experience affects marriage and other intimate relationships, re-entry into peer groups, and employment and insurance. The issues of employment and loss of insurance are usually not applicable to older women, however no literature was found to describe other consequences experienced by older women who survive cancer. Surviving cancer brings with it an entire new realm of circumstances and issues. "There is no moment of cure, but rather an evolution of survival beginning with diagnosis" (Quigley, 1989, p. 63). How does this experience affect the cancer patient's quality of life? More specifically, how does this impact the older woman?

By assessing the quality of life of older women, one might determine if acceptable outcomes have occurred in the treatment process (Foreman & Kleinpell, 1990). Questions for researchers to ask include, what exactly is quality of life, and is it different for the older woman than it is for the younger woman? Early research in this area focused on variables related strictly to functional status; in other words, if a person could carry out activities of daily living, then researchers assumed the patient had psychosocial well-being (Quigley, 1989). Information based solely on functional status could provide a skewed view of the older woman's quality of life. The decrease in physiological capacity that comes with aging often alters an older woman's functional status, which may or may not decrease her quality of life. Recent research in this area has expanded to include such issues as psychological state, interpersonal relationships, and personal well-being (Quigley, 1989; Foreman & Kleinpell, 1990).

REDUCING THE RISK OF CANCER IN THE OLDER WOMAN: GOALS FOR THE 21ST CENTURY

Healthy People 2000 (1990), a report compiled by more than 300 health related organizations, discusses the state of Americans' health today and goals toward a healthier society by the year 2000. In the area of cancer, the report sets forth objectives that target those areas of prevention and detection that exhibit the greatest potential in reducing the incidence, morbidity, and mortality of cancer. The priority areas include reduction in cigarette smoking, dietary changes, and greater utilization of early detection mechanisms.

Goals specific to smoking include slowing the rise in lung cancer deaths and reducing the prevalence of cigarette smoking to no more than 15 percent in individuals 20 years of age and older. This would represent a 30 percent reduction for women (Healthy People 2000, 1990).

Nutritional goals involve the reduction of fat intake to 30 percent of total daily calories with 10 percent or less coming from saturated fats, and increasing consumption of complex carbohydrates to five or more servings of fruits and vegetables per day, and six or more servings of grain products. For women in the United States, this would represent about a 30 percent and a 50 percent increase, respectively (Healthy People 2000, 1990).

Enhancing the use of early detection measures can decrease the mortality rates of cancer. The multiple goals in this area obviously target both men and women. Goals specifically related to the older woman include the use of breast examination, mammography, and the Pap test. Clinical research indicates that for the woman 50 years of age and older, the use of mammography and clinical breast examination can decrease mortality as much as 30 percent. With this in mind, the goals set forth in the report call for increasing to at least 60 percent the number of women age 50 and over who have had both a clinical breast exam and mammography within the previous one to two years. This would be approximately a 42 percent increase for woman age 70 and older. Though younger women are diagnosed with cervical cancer more frequently, the stage of the disease at the time of diagnosis in older women is usually much more advanced. Hence, the goal for this area sets forth having at least 95 percent of all women over the age of 18 receive a Pap test until 85 percent are being tested within the preceding one to three years. This should reduce mortality as much as 75 percent (Healthy People 2000, 1990).

Because factors such as lifestyle and environment can increase one's risk for cancer, for the older woman in the 21st century to be healthy, the medical community must take steps now to adequately educate and provide health services for all women regardless of age, race, or economic status. Coupled with this, each woman must take charge of her health as she is able and thus reduce her risks of acquiring cancer (Healthy People 2000, 1990).

STRATEGIES FOR LIVING WITH CANCER

When considering how to promote healthy and productive living in the older woman with cancer, it is necessary to recognize the importance of coping skills and support systems. Literature dealing with individuals suffering from chronic illnesses identify hope as an essential element to adapt to the changes that occur during the course of illness (Raleigh, 1992). In a study designed to determine factors that influence effective coping, hope was identified as a primary element determining an individual's ability to cope with a life-threatening illness (Hung, 1975). Research by Herth (1989) indicates that there is a significant relationship between a cancer patient's level of hope and level of effective coping responses. In conjunction with the need for hope, the need and importance of a strong support system is consistently reported in the literature (Raleigh, 1992; Herth, 1989; O'Conner, Wicker & Germino, 1990; and Krause, 1991). What does this mean for the older woman with cancer? Strategies for "healthy living" even though diagnosed with cancer include maximizing one's strengths and fostering a sense of hope and purpose despite the threat of serious illness.

The issue of rehabilitation is a relatively new and untapped strategy for living with the cancer experience. Though recognized as an essential component in the treatment of cancer, very few programs have been developed to date that provide for the rehabilitation needs of the older woman (Johnson & Kelly, 1990). One such experience however, is reported by Johnson and Kelly (1990), in which a multifaceted program of rehabilitation was developed for women diagnosed with breast cancer. This program emphasized wellness and optimal functioning regardless of the presence of cancer, and fostered the development of attitudes such as hope, independence, courage and determination. Participants in the program reported experiencing an increase in their own confidence level in dealing with the disease and its challenges, and a stronger sense of social support.

The task of healthy living for an older woman with cancer is challenging but attainable. Health care workers must be sensitive to issues such as quality of life and survivorship, prevention, coping skills, support systems and cancer rehabilitation as they assist the older woman in assessing her options and formulating a plan in order to live a healthy and productive life, despite the presence of disease.

The Role of the Health Care Provider

Given the characteristics of successful adaptation to living with cancer, a logical questions is: How can these behaviors be learned or enhanced? There is support in the literature that health care workers can teach, enhance, or support these behaviors. One strong theme that emerged in the successful adaptation behaviors is the notion of hope; having it and maintaining it (Hickey, 1986 & Owen, 1989). According to Owen hope can be facilitated by health care providers. Specific measures suggested are assisting the woman to identify reasons for living. One means of accomplishing this is by assisting women with goal setting. Depending on the situation this might be immediate goals (those activities related to survival); short term goals, 3-6 months (a short trip); or long term goals (completing a project). Many women find hope through religion. Health care providers can support women as they seek to maintain contacts with their organized religions or to reestablish contact. Humor can be another avenue for maintaining hope and one that can be introduced in daily contacts or in a more organized way through use of humorous movies or videos.

Another suggestion for supporting coping strategies is through use of social support systems. Family and friends are obvious sources of social support. However, systems of support can be developed for the older woman with cancer. One common way is through support groups. The American Cancer Society has several support groups: CanSurmount, I Can Cope, and Reach to Recovery. Groups can be used for discussing common emotions, teaching methods of reducing stress, and teaching and sharing ways of taking control in a situation that may seem out of control (Fredette & Beattie, 1986). Support groups need to be previewed by health care providers before blanket recommendations are made. Pillon (1991) suggests that a single support group may not meet everyone's needs and notes that different subgroups may be needed based on the participants' age and stage of cancer.

Health care providers can further support women with cancer through giving information, answering questions, and clarifying misconceptions. This can be done one-to-one as recommended by Welch-McCaffrey (1986) when working with women over 65 or as an education component of a support group. In addition to information about the disease and treatment, information about available community resources can assist women with cancer to cope.

An additional area of information that can enhance a woman's control even as she enters the terminal stage of cancer is in regards to hospice care. The goal of hospice care is to enable persons with cancer to be alert and pain free and to spend their final days in dignity and quality either in their own home or in a homelike environment. This goal supports a woman's choices even if the outcome is not cure and survival (Mayer, 1992).

An attitude change that can be supported by health care workers is to shift from the idea of the cancer "victim" to the cancer survivor (Mayer, 1992). This may seem like semantics but words carry power and self-esteem can be enhanced or detracted by other peoples' attitudes. Further enhancement of self-esteem may be supported through encouraging women to exercise. Nelson (1991) reports that women who had had breast cancer and practiced more health promoting behaviors (walking, stretching, aerobics) also had higher ratings of self-esteem.

CONCLUSION

The risk of getting cancer increases with age. Prevention would be the preferred course for decreasing the numbers of new cases, however in many instances the exact cause of the cancer is unknown. That leaves early detection as the next best course of action. For the woman over 65 there are problems with early detection: misperceptions of the women themselves, low usage of early detection tests, lack of programs developed specifically with the needs of the older woman in mind, and disinterest by health professionals in developing programs suitable for this age group, to mention a few. If a woman over 65 gets cancer, there are also problems with treatment. Therapies may be limited because of age bias or because of the presence of other chronic illness. Even in survivorship there are concerns, many of them centered around the fact that very little is known about the female cancer survivor over 65 and how survivorship affects her quality of life. It is evident that some women with cancer lead productive lives. Some of the attributes are known:

maintaining hope as a means of coping and strong support systems; there are more strategies to be elucidated through study. There are community programs and strategies that health care providers can implement. Research to establish the effectiveness of these programs along with issues surrounding quality of life, survivorship and treatment is needed. It is apparent that when it comes to issues related to women, aging, and cancer there are more questions than answers.

REFERENCES

American Cancer Society. (1992). *Cancer Facts & Figures*. Atlanta, Georgia: Author.

American Cancer Society. (1992). *Estimated New Cancer Cases*. Atlanta, Georgia: Department of Epidemiology and Statistics.

Blesch, K.S., & Prohaska, T.R. (1991). Cervical cancer screening in older women. *Cancer Nursing, 14*(3), 141-147.

Boarini, J. (1987). Gastrointestinal malignancies: colon and rectum. In S.L. Groenwald (Ed.), *Cancer Nursing Principles and Practice* (pp. 544-557). Boston: Jones and Bartlett.

Celentano, D. (1989). Early detection of cervical cancer in elderly women. In R. Yancik, & J. Yates (Eds.), *Cancer in the Elderly* (pp. 15-27). New York: Springer Publ. Co.

Celentano, D.D., Shapiro, S., & Weisman, C.S. (1982). Cancer preventive screening behavior among elderly women. *Preventive Medicine, 11*(4), 454-463.

Centers for Disease Control. (1987). Provisional estimates from the national health survey supplement of cancer control, United States. *Morbidity and Mortality Weekly Reports, 37*(27), 417-419.

Clinical Practice Committee: American Geriatrics Society. (1989). Screening for breast cancer in elderly women. *Journal of American Geriatrics Society, 37*(9), 883-884.

Clinical Practice Committee: American Geriatrics Society. (1989). Screening for cervical carcinoma in elderly women. *Journal of American Geriatrics Society, 37*(9), 885-887.

Department of Health and Human Services. (1990). *Healthy People 2000*. (DHHS Publication No. (PHS) 91-50212). Washington, DC: U. S. Government Printing Office.

Donegan, W.L. (1983). Treatment of breast cancer in the elderly. In R. Yancik, P. P. Carbone, W.B. Patterson, K. Steele, & W. D. Terry (Eds.). *Perspectives on Prevention and Treatment of Cancer in the Elderly* (pp. 83-96). New York: Raven Press.

Dow, K.J. (1990). The enduring seasons of survival. *Oncology Nursing Forum, 17*(4), 511-516.

Elpern, E.H. (1987). Bronchogenic malignancies. In S.L. Groenwald (Ed.), *Cancer Nursing Principles and Practice* (pp. 470-488). Boston: Jones and Bartlett.

Foreman, M.D., & Kleinpell, R. (1990). Assessing the quality of life of elderly persons. *Seminars in Oncology Nursing, 6*(4), 292-297.

Fredette, S.L., & Beattie, H.M. (1986). Living with cancer. *Cancer Nursing, 9*(6), 308-316.

Garfinkel, L., & Stellman, S.D. (1988). Smoking and lung cancer in women: Findings in a prospective study. *Cancer Research, 48*(23), 6951-6955.

Goodman, M.S. (1987). Breast malignancies. In S.L. Groenwald (Ed.), *Cancer Nursing Principles and Practice* (pp. 442-469). Boston: Jones and Bartlett.

Greenfield, S., Aronow, H.V., Gtanz, P.A., & Elashoff, R.M. (1989). The effect of age in the management of elderly cancer patients. In R. Yancik & J.W. Yates (Eds.). *Cancer in the Elderly: Approaches to Early Detection and Treatment* (pp. 55-70). New York: Springer.

Harris, R.P., Fletcher, S.W., Gonzalez, J.J., Lannin, D.R., Degan, D., Earp, J.A., & Clark, R. (1991). Mammography and age: Are we targeting the wrong women? *Cancer, 67*(7), 2010-2014.

Herth, K.A. (1989). The relationship between level of hope and level of coping response and other variables in patients with cancer. *Oncology Nursing Forum, 16*(1), 67-72.

Hickey, S.S. (1986). Enabling hope. *Cancer Nursing, 9*(3), 133-137.

Hoffman, B. (1989). Cancer survivors at work: Job problems and illegal discrimination. *Oncology Nursing Forum, 16*(1), 39-43.

Hung, A. (1975). Coping behavior of patients and their families to life-threatening illness (brain tumor). Doctoral Dissertation, School of Social Work, Columbia University. *Dissertation Abstracts International, 39*(1), 469A.

Johnson, J.B., & Kelly, A.W. (1990). A multifaceted rehabilitation program for women with cancer. *Oncology Nursing Forum, 17*(5), 691-695.

Kelsey, J.L., & Gammon, M.D. (1991). The epidemiology of breast cancer. *CA-A Cancer Journal for Clinicians, 41*(3), 146-165.

Krause, K. (1991). Contracting cancer and coping with it. *Cancer Nursing, 14*(5), 240-245.

Loescher, L.J., Clark, L., Atwood, J.R., Leigh, S., & Lamb, G. (1990). Impact of the cancer experience on long-term survivors. *Oncology Nursing Forum, 17*(2), 223-229.

Luckman, J., & Sorensen, K.C. (1987). *Medical-Surgical Nursing: A Pathophysiological Approach,* 3rd. ed. Philadelphia: W.B. Saunders.

Mayer, D.K. (1992). The healthcare implications of cancer rehabilitation in the twenty-first century. *Oncology Nursing Forum, 19*(1), 23-27.

McCaffrey Boyle, D., Engelking, C., Smith Blesch, K., Dodge, J., Sarna, L., & Weinrich, S. (1992). ONS position paper on cancer and aging. *Oncology Nursing Forum, 19*(6), 913-933.

Mettlin, C., & Dodd, G.D. (1991). The American Cancer Society guidelines for the cancer-related checkup: An update. *Ca-A Cancer Journal for Clinicians, 41*(5), 279-282.

Miller, N.J., & Pazdur, M. (1987). Gynecologic malignancies. In S.L. Groenwald (Ed.), *Cancer Nursing Principles and Practice* (pp. 558-591). Boston: Jones and Bartlett.

Nelson, J.P. (1991). Perceived health, self-esteem, health habits, and perceived benefits and barriers to exercise in women who have and who have not experienced stage I breast cancer. *Oncology Nursing Forum, 19*(7), 1191-1197.

O'Conner, A.P., Wicker, C.A., & Germino, B.B. (1990). Understanding the cancer patient's search for meaning. *Cancer Nursing, 13*(3), 167-175.

Owen, D.C. (1989). Nurses perspectives on the meaning of hope in patients with cancer: A qualitative study. *Oncology Nursing Forum, 16*(1), 75-79.

Pathak, D.R., Samet, J.M., Humble, C.G., & Skipper, B.J. (1986). Determinants of lung cancer risk in cigarette smokers in New Mexico. *Journal of the National Cancer Institute, 76*(4), 597-604.

Pillon, L.R., & Gayle, J. (1991). An 11-year evaluation of a living with cancer program. *Oncology Nursing Forum, 18*(4), 707-711.

Quigley, K.M. (1989). The adult cancer survivor: psychosocial consequences of cure. *Seminars in Oncology Nursing, 5*(1), 63-69.

Raleigh, E.O.H. (1992). Sources of hope in chronic illness. *Oncology Nursing Forum, 19*(3), 443-448.

Ries, L.A.G., Hankey, B.F., Miller, B.A. et al. (1991). *Cancer statistics review, 1973-1988,* NIH Pub. No. 91-2789, Bethesda, MD: National Cancer Institute, 1991.

Rimer, B., Jones, W., Wilson, C., Bennett, D., & Engstrom, P. (1983). Planning a cancer control program for older citizens. *The Gerontologist, 23*(4), 384-389.

Schmale, A., Morrow, G.R., Schmitt, M.H., Adler, L.M., Enelow, A., Murawski, B.J., & Gates, C. (1983). Well-being of cancer survivors. *Psychosomatic Medicine, 45*(2), 163-169.

Simon, J.B. (1985). Occult blood screening for colorectal cancer: A critical review. *Gastroenterology, 88*(3), 820-837.

Weinrich, S.P. (1990). Predictors of older adults' participation in fecal occult blood screening. *Oncology Nursing Forum, 17*(5), 715-720.

Welch-McCaffrey, D. (1986). To teach or not to teach? Overcoming barriers to patient education in geriatric oncology. *Oncology Nursing Forum, 13*(4), 25-30.

Welch-McCaffrey, D.W., Hoffman, B., Leigh, S.A., Loescher, L.J., & Meyskens, F.L. (1989). Surviving adult cancer. Part 2: Psychosocial implications. *Annals of Internal Medicine, 111*(6), 517-524.

Winawer, S., Schotenfeld, P., & Sherlock, P. (1985). Screening for colorectal cancer: The issues. *Gastroenterology, 88*(3), 841-844.

Yancik, R., Kessler, L., & Yates, J.W. (1988). The elderly population opportunities for cancer prevention and detection. *Cancer, 62*(8), 1823-1828.

Alzheimer's Disease and Older Women

Elaine Souder, PhD, RN

SUMMARY. The graying of America suggests that dementia will become "the epidemic of the 21st century." First described in 1907, Alzheimer's Disease (AD) accounts for an estimated two-thirds of all dementia. AD currently has no cure, thus causing a major drain on health care and family resources. Compared to men, women are uniquely affected by AD due to their gender-associated increased risk, longer life span, and roles as caregivers within families and institutions. Living successfully with dementia requires medical and behavioral interventions to manage disruptive symptoms, knowledge to optimize environmental conditions, and caregiver support and savvy to avoid burnout. Strategies for maximizing functioning in older women living with AD are provided.

Demographic trends suggest that dementia will become "the epidemic of the 21st century" (Bachman, Wolf, Linn, Knoefel, Cobb, Belanger et al., 1992, p. 21) and represents a critical health care concern as the population of older adults increases. The old-old (> 85 years of age) subgroup represents the fastest growing segment of the U.S. population and has increased 33 percent from 1980 to 1990 (Cohen & Van Nostrand, 1992). An analysis of 47 prevalence studies concluded that the prevalence of dementia has doubled every 5.1 years (Jorm, Korten, & Henderson, 1987).

Dementia refers not to a specific disease but to an umbrella of disorders that share characteristics of acquired cognitive dysfunc-

---

Elaine Souder is affiliated with the College of Nursing and Medicine, University of Arkansas for Medical Sciences, Little Rock, AR 72205.

[Haworth co-indexing entry note]: "Alzheimer's Disease and Older Women." Souder, Elaine. Co-published simultaneously in the *Journal of Women & Aging* (The Haworth Press, Inc.) Vol. 5, No. 3/4, 1993, pp. 139-154; and: *Women and Healthy Aging: Living Productively in Spite of It All* (ed: J. Dianne Garner, and Alice A. Young), The Haworth Press, Inc., 1993, pp. 139-154. Multiple copies of this article/chapter may be purchased from The Haworth Document Delivery Center [1-800-3-HAWORTH; 9:00 a.m.-5:00 p.m. (EST)].

139

tion, accompanied by impaired functioning in everyday activities (APA, 1987). Dr. Alois Alzheimer first described Alzheimer's Disease (AD) in 1907, and it now accounts for an estimated two thirds of all dementia in the U.S. (Schoenberg, Kokmen, & Okazaki, 1987) and stands as the fourth leading cause of death in the Western world (Khatchaturian, 1987; Reisberg, 1983).

Dementia places an immense burden on families, institutions, and society. More than 70 percent of those with less severe disease receive care at home at an estimated cost of $12,000 annually per family. Because the average duration of AD spans eight years, however, most patients eventually are institutionalized. Currently, the total cost for care, lost productivity, and early death of Alzheimer patients stands at an estimated $90 billion annually (NIA, 1992).

Dementia uniquely affects women for four reasons. First, women live longer than men (Cohen & Van Nostrand, 1992) thus making them at increased risk for dementia in later life. Second, the incidence of dementia is higher in women than in men, even when age is controlled. In a recent Framingham Study report that used strict clinical criteria, the overall rate of dementia for men was 30.5/1000, compared to 48.2/1000 in women. The gender difference was striking, however, in AD. Women had a reported rate of 30.1/1000, compared to 11.7/1000 in men (Bachman et al., 1992). Third, because American women traditionally have assumed the caregiver role, women are more likely than men to provide care for spouses, parents, and parents-in-law who have dementia (Gatz, Bengtson, & Blum, 1990). Fourth, more women than men provide direct nursing care to patients with dementia in nursing homes and hospitals.

This paper will discuss the causes, disease process, diagnosis, and offer suggestions for living productively and maximizing functioning after a diagnosis of AD has been made.

OVERVIEW OF CAUSES

The official manual of the American Psychiatric Association contains an entry of Primary Degenerative Dementia (PPD) of the Alzheimer Type, which is characterized by a slow onset, progressive deterioration, and exclusion of all other known specific causes

(APA, 1987). PPD and vascular or multi-infarct dementia (MID) account for more than 70 percent of all cases of cognitive impairment in old age (Nussbaum, Treves, & Korczyn, 1992).

Researchers have developed many theories concerning the causes of AD in the past decade. Part of the difficulty lies in elucidating the causes versus the effects of the brain dysfunction. The etiology of AD may involve a genetic defect on chromosome 21, other mono- or poly-genic defects, nongenetic agents, or a combination of environmental and genetic factors (St. George-Hyslop, Haines, Farrer, Polinsky, Van Broeckhoven, Goate et al., 1990). More specific hypotheses have implicated infective agents, metabolic dysfunction, neurochemical deficits, and changes in blood-brain barriers (Khachaturian, 1991).

Several risk factors for AD include increased age, head-injury, Down's syndrome, and family history of AD (Mortimer, Van Duijn, Chandra et al., 1991). With the exception of safety practices to decrease head injury in automobile accidents and a ban on boxing, none of the identified risk factors are modifiable with current knowledge (Rabins, 1992).

Ample evidence points to heterogeneity in AD. In a recent review of clinical and biological research reporting heterogeneity, Ritchie and Touchon (1992) described three models to summarize the quantitative and qualitative differences documented within the Alzheimer population. First, they presented some evidence for a phase model, which assumes a homogenous global and orderly progressive deterioration. A second model suggests that variable patterns of deterioration may evolve according to individual neurobiological compensatory processes. The strongest scientific support suggests that heterogeneity exists due to sub-types of the disease, although current knowledge cannot define the underlying biological mechanisms responsible for the functional impairment patterns in these sub-groups. Khatchaturian (1987) suggests that a number of etiological factors may cause various disorders that are expressed through a final pathway, which we observe and diagnose as AD. Additional research including longitudinal studies must occur to consider cohort effects and the normal variations in elderly cognitive performance.

DIAGNOSIS

Clinicians must conduct a thorough diagnostic workup in each case to detect underlying treatable disorders and potentially reversible conditions that mimic AD. Misdiagnosis of potentially reversible conditions ranging from depression to drug toxicity can lead to inappropriate treatment including institutionalization. Additionally, an early and thorough workup will enable appropriate planning in which the affected woman can participate.

Jorm, Fratiglioni, and Winblad (1993) discuss two separate and difficult steps involved in the diagnosis of dementia. The first is to differentiate dementia from the continuum of normal aging presentations; the second is to differentiate the diseases that produce a dementia. Diagnosis of AD may be considered a diagnosis by exclusion. Due to the lack of a biological marker, experts frequently refer to the disease as dementia of the Alzheimer type (DAT) or probable AD (Morris & Rubin, 1991).

Major sets of criteria have been developed to assist in the diagnosis of AD. One of the most widely used was developed by The National Institute of Neurological and Communicative Disorders and Stroke-Alzheimer's Disease and Related Disorders Association (NINCDS-ADRDA) Work Group (McKhann, Drachman, Folstein, Katzman, Price, & Stadlan, 1984). The NINCDS-ADRDA criteria, categorized as "possible," "probable," and "definite" AD, have high accuracy rates of diagnosis (Forette, Henry, & Orgogozo, 1989). The second set of criteria were published in the DSM-III-R (APA, 1987). These are currently under revision and will be part of the DSM-IV.

The definitive diagnosis of AD requires histopathologic evidence of a particular distribution and density of senile plaques and neurofibrillary tangles, the microscopic hallmarks obtainable only at autopsy or by brain biopsy. Clinicians rarely perform brain biopsy due to the associated high risk of infection. Of concern, however, is a recent study of physician practices in the diagnosis of AD. Seventy-five percent of the physicians did not use either the DSM-III or NINCDS-ADRDA diagnostic criteria (Somerfield, Weisman, Ury, Chase, & Folstein, 1991).

A recent effort reflecting input from experts in many major research centers has resulted in a new set of diagnostic criteria developed by the Consortium to Establish a Registry for Alzheimer's

Disease (CERAD) (Morris, Heyman, Mohs, Hughes, Van Belle, Fillenbaum et al., 1989). This group is seeking to standardize assessment and promote a uniform evaluation in the diagnostic workup of AD, improve accuracy and efficiency in diagnosing the individual patient, and facilitate research.

The differential diagnosis of AD includes MID, the second most common form of dementia. A series of small infarcts in the brain, typically related to long-standing hypertension and/or diabetes cause MID. MID and AD appear to coexist in approximately 15 percent of individuals with dementia. A demarcated, "step-wise," or patchy deterioration that results from successive infarcts typifies MID, in contrast to the more gradual, global pattern seen in AD. Uneven and selective mental deterioration also characterize MID. Unlike most dementias, MID is potentially preventable through early detection and treatment of hypertension and heart disease. Dementia also occurs in 15-50 percent of cases of Parkinson's disease, normal pressure hydrocephalus, Creutzfeldt-Jakob disease, Huntington's chorea, Pick's disease, and diffuse encephalopathies of uncertain origin, and some cases of AIDS (Wells, 1985).

Misdiagnosis of AD may occur in reversible medical and psychiatric conditions, such as delirium, electrolyte disturbance, hypothyroidism, and depression. In addition, physicians frequently underdiagnose alcohol and prescription drug abuse in elderly females, also contributing to the misdiagnosis of AD (in press). Although many researches have paid attention to these "pseudodementias," Clarefield (1988) reviewed numerous studies and reported an overall potentially reversible rate of only 13.2 percent. Increasingly, research suggests that conditions formerly thought reversible forms of dementia are, in fact, early presentations of eventual dementia.

Lowenthal and Nadeau (1991) suggest that polypharmacy, in the context of normal aging and multiple systemic illnesses, constitutes the "third strike" and can send the patient out of the game. Drug toxicity can occur when patients mix over-the-counter with prescribed medications, alter the prescribed dose, self-medicate, or use a variety of drugs from different sources without adequate communication among prescribers. Because age-related changes also alter physiological responses of drugs, previously prescribed medications may need dosage adjustment to obtain usual benefits. Drugs at high risk of causing cognitive impairment include psychotropics, drugs with anticholinergic properties, certain groups of antihypertensive agents, cardiac drugs, anticonvulsants, and sedative-hypnotics (Lowenthal & Nadeau, 1991).

State of the art neuroimaging techniques can serve as useful adjuncts in the diagnostic process; however, experts consider none definitive at this time. Computed axial tomographs (CT) and magnetic resonance imaging (MRI) show brain structures, identify potentially treatable causes of impairment, such as tumor, or normal pressure hydrocephalus, and document ventricular and sulcal enlargement commonly noted in AD. Although atrophy of the brain is easily documented in AD, it also exists to varying degrees in normal aging. Single photon emission tomography (SPECT) and positron emission tomography (PET) differ from the anatomical scans because they reveal brain physiology. Because brain physiology may change before the anatomical structures, SPECT and PET scans may show decreased blood flow or metabolism even though CT or MRI scans appear normal. Despite great interest and aspirations of neuroimagers, PET will likely remain a research instrument. Experts predict that SPECT, however, will become increasingly popular in assessment of dementia (Guze, Hoffman, Baxter, Mazziotta, & Phelps, 1991).

SYMPTOMS AND DISEASE PROGRESSION

In a review of AD, Morris and Rubin (1991) found two patterns of decline. More than half progressed from mild to severe illness over a three-year period while the remaining patients had courses of variable deterioration. The reason for this difference remains unknown although various theories have emerged. In their study, 30 percent had died within five years, and 73 percent of those alive at five years were living in institutions (Morris & Rubin, 1991). The lifespan typically ranges from ten to fourteen years from diagnosis.

The literature on AD frequently refers to early, middle, and late stages of the disease (Gwyther, 1985). The first stage lasts two to four years and covers the period leading up to and including the diagnosis. During this period, the individual experiences confusion about places, loses things, shows poor judgment, and exhibits difficulty handling money and bills. In addition, the person may have mood and personality changes and lose initiative. Morris and Rubin (1991) note that aphasia and difficulties with reading and comprehension occur in approximately one third of patients with mild AD.

The informants of 200 patients meeting CERAD criteria cited memory problems (98.5%) that typically interfere with daily living functions in mild AD (Morris & Rubin, 1991). At least 75 percent of the informants also mentioned disorientation and impaired activities of daily living. They less frequently identified personality change (47.5%) and language impairment (41.5%). A number of AD studies have shown significant impairment of odor recognition, odor identification, or odor memory (Doty, Reyes, & Gregor, 1987; Rezek, 1987). These abnormalities apparently exist very early in AD and may be among the earliest symptoms of the disorder.

Psychiatric symptoms are quite common and have received less attention than memory impairment (Flint, 1991). Depression exists in about 25 percent of AD patients and, if treated, will reduce excess disability even though cognitive function will not improve (Kramer & Reifler, 1992). Delusions, which may occur in any stage of AD, may be simple, complex, persecutory, grandiose, or accompaniments to neuropsychological deficits (Cummings, Millet, Hill, & Neshkes, 1987). Although in need of further research, delusions may represent dysfunction secondary to the disease process. Misidentifications of television or mirror images as well as familiar persons may be a type of delusion related to neurological deficit (Burns, 1992). A second psychiatric symptom, hallucinations, may occur in visual, olfactory, or auditory forms. Rabins reported 49 percent of caregivers indicated the presence of hallucinations (Rabins, Mace, & Lucas, 1982), a finding supported by a number of additional studies.

In the second stage, which lasts from two to ten years, the Alzheimer's patient has increased memory loss and confusion, difficulty recognizing friends and family members, restlessness as the day progresses, muscle twitches/jerking, word-finding problems, suspiciousness, irritability, crying, loss of impulse control, reluctance to bathe, weight change, difficulty organizing thoughts, and repetitive statements or movements. Family caregivers may have difficulty managing the disruption of wake/sleep cycle and wandering.

The terminal phase consists of several years in which the individual has weight loss, inability to talk or care for self, bowel and bladder incontinence, difficulty with swallowing, increased sleep, and loss of awareness of environment and self, ending in death due to sepsis or malnutrition (Harrell, 1991).

TREATMENT OPTIONS AND ISSUES

Because the road of progressive deterioration may take many turns, it is advisable to have the assistance of an interested and knowledgeable physician to monitor medical needs. Many family caregivers have verbalized that physicians seemed disinterested after making a diagnosis of AD. If the patient or family members are uncomfortable with the quality of physician contacts, they should consider finding someone with whom rapport and caring interactions are possible.

Whitehouse (1991) has described short, intermediate, and long-term strategies to manage symptoms of AD. From the short-term perspective, physicians can use medications to treat cognitive symptoms as well as behavioral disturbances that frequently occur. They can implement symptomatic pharmacologic treatment of specific symptoms such as agitation, confusion, or depression as part of an overall treatment program (Katzman & Jackson, 1991). Physicians also can employ drug trials and cognitive enhancers (Calvani & Carta, 1991; Jarvik, Berg, Bartus, Heston, Leith, Phelps et al., 1990). Whitehouse (1991) notes that the FDA is experiencing political pressure to relax efficacy standards for new medications to treat AD. Scientists are conducting studies of a dozen medications in the U.S. In addition to drugs such as tacrine designed to stimulate single neurotransmitter systems, scientists are investigating compounds that stimulate multiple neurotransmitter systems.

Intermediate term strategies can include pharmacologic agents designed to prevent death and maximize functioning of nerve cells. Most of these are still in developmental stages. Long-term strategies require increased knowledge of the underlying pathophysiology of AD, and may take the form of exogenous neuronal transplants in brains, genetic alteration, or medications to slow the progression of the disease (Whitehouse, 1991).

Although AD affects both cognition and behavior, scientists know little about effective management of behavior problems. Several nurse researcher groups have launched research programs focused on management of behavioral problems. Beck and colleagues have developed interventions to maximize independence in dressing behaviors (Beck, 1990; Beck, Heacock, Mercer, & Walton, 1992). Van Ort and Phillips (1992) reported successful behavioral interventions in eating behaviors of demented individuals in nursing homes. Teri, Rabins, Whitehouse, Berg, Reisberg, Sunderland et al. (1992) have clearly identified the imperative need, current knowledge, and future directions in managing behavioral disturbances in AD.

I have known many women who have volunteered to participate in a dementia research program, either as a patient or as a caregiver. They verbalized that through research activity and involvement, they hoped to advance science to help others with the disease (Souder, 1992). I also observed that participation in research provided a way for them to gain some meaning to the experience and to learn more about the disease that was affecting their lives so deeply.

STRATEGIES TO MAXIMIZE FUNCTIONING

Living successfully with dementia requires medical and behavioral interventions to manage disruptive symptoms, knowledge to optimize environmental conditions, and caregiver support and savvy to avoid burnout. In addition, experts recommend paying attention to nutrition, exercise, and lifestyle factors to maintain healthy physical aging.

Fabiszewski (1986) suggests that the goals in helping someone live with dementia consist of promoting enjoyment and pleasure in life, facilitating participation, promoting comfort, maintaining dignity and fostering feelings of safety and security. In addition, the caregiver should strive to eliminate excess disability.

Following a diagnosis of dementia, the individual and family or significant others need to address several issues. First, if employed, the family and the individual need to consider when to terminate employment to minimize jeopardy to dignity and financial stress. In some cases, the affected person can continue to work at the same place of employment in a less demanding role. A family member or significant other should have durable power of attorney to make future decisions for the patient if necessary. One spousal caregiver told me of a tragic situation in which her husband, after devoting his entire adulthood to building a successful business, sold it for $5,000 to his business partner. The wife was initiating legal proceedings to reverse the decision, but that recourse carried significant stress and costs. Before cognitive abilities further deteriorate, the patient should share preferences regarding institutional care in the event that it is required. In the early stage of illness, the patient also should write or update a will and develop a living will that conveys one's wishes regarding the extent of life sustaining treatment.

The woman with or caring for someone with AD should strive to decrease five stressors that can accentuate behavioral symptoms (Hall, 1988). These include changes in routine, demanding environment, excess stimuli, fatigue, and physical stressors that accompany physical illness. Therefore, the family or significant others should offer a structured daily routine that does not vary from day to day, an environment free of excessive or distracting stimulation, and predictable and simple routines (Weiner, 1991). The caregiver can decrease stress by offering a narrow choice of clothes, food, and activities.

Environmental cues can help maximize independent functioning in a familiar environment. In one home, the healthy spouse had placed a picture of herself on a card with her work phone number printed in large numbers by the telephone. Caregivers can place simple figures or photographs on cupboard doors to remind the person of the location of frequently-used items.

A number of environmental changes can help decrease stress. Koenig-Coste quoted in Kent (1992) suggests using bright, solid colors with contrast to assist with depth perception and avoid over-stimulation. She also recommends minimizing environmental noise and clutter and removing throw rugs to decrease risk of injury.

A major goal of care at home centers on maximizing patient functioning while preventing accidents. In the early stages, AD patients are prone to traffic accidents due to definite mental impairment, slow reaction time, confusion about meaning of road signs and traffic lights, difficulty gauging distance between vehicles, being easily distracted, and becoming lost. Later in the disease, accidents also can occur as repeated falls and personal injuries due to medical conditions, medication side effects, and environmental hazards (difficulty gauging height of door thresholds, steps, curbs, and other barriers). Caregivers should highlight edges in bright colors. Fire and electrical hazards pose threats due to poor memory or easy distractibility. Bathroom dangers include failure to turn off the water and gauge water temperature. Other threats include accidental poisoning and under or over medication with prescription drugs. Caregivers should remove toxic or hazardous cleaning supplies from home. To increase safety in individuals who wander, change locks, child-proof door handles, establish an alarm door system and provide an ID on bracelet (Tackenberg, 1992).

In addition to environmental issues, interpersonal communications can facilitate emotional security and self-esteem. The Alzheimer's Association (1985) recommends that caregivers pay attention to their tone of voice and nonverbal communication and avoid talking in abstractions and asking questions when possible. Experts also advise that families refrain from confronting their loved ones with cognitive limitations (Weiner, Bruhn, Svetlik, Tintner, & Hom, 1991). Gwyther (1991) advises caregivers to respond to the feeling behind the words. Frequently, when a person continually asks for someone deceased, it is effective to respond to the feeling of missing someone special rather than providing information that the person is deceased.

The caregiver plays a critical role in the well-being of the person with dementia. Research has amply demonstrated that caregivers, as a group, are at risk for depression, burn-out, and impaired health (Anthony-Bergstone, Zarit, & Gatz, 1988; George & Gwyther, 1986). The local and national chapters of the Alzheimer's Disease and Related Disorders Association (ADRDA), offer hot lines, support groups, and newsletters that provide announcements of classes and lectures, suggestions for dealing with problematic behaviors, and news of the latest research and legislative efforts to benefit those living with dementia. Meeting one's own needs becomes difficult as caregiving demands increase, and the individual caregiver must find sources of enjoyment and diversion to balance the stressful demands. In an unforgettable interview, one woman emphasized that she could cope with the caregiving as long as she had periodic breaks from the responsibilities by visiting Las Vegas with friends. When the caregiving demands mounted, she remembered and anticipated her next visit to Las Vegas.

CONCLUSIONS

AD poses formidable challenges to older women, health care providers, scientists, and society. Although AD currently has no cure, women living with AD can maximize functioning by effective planning for the future, maintaining physical health, decreasing environmental demands and stressors, avoiding fatigue, and modifying the environment to promote independent functioning and safety.

RESOURCES

Alzheimer's Disease and Related Disorders Association (ADRDA)
70 East Lake Street
Chicago, IL 60601
1-800-621-0379
Illinois: 1-800-572-6037

National Institute of Aging Alzheimer's Disease Education and Referral Center (ADEAR)
#NIAC, P.O. Box 8250
Silver Spring, MD 20907
1-800-438-4380

The Agency for Health Care Policy and Research (AHCPR) is developing new *Clinical Practice Guideline,* for publication in 1993:
AHCPR Publications Clearinghouse
P.O. Box 8547
Silver Spring, MD 20907
1-800-358-9295

Books for the Caregiver

Gwyther, L. (1985). *Care of Alzheimer patients: A Manual for the Nursing Home Staff*, $5.00 (Excellent reference for home care).

Cohen, D. & Eisdorfer, C. (1986). *Loss of self.* New York: New American Library, $7.95.

Aronson, M.K. (Ed.) (1988). *Understanding Alzheimer's Disease.* Chicago: Alzheimer's Disease and Related Disorders Association, $15.95.

Mace, N. & Rabins, P. (1991). *The 36-Hour Day.* Baltimore: Johns Hopkins University Press (A popular guide now available in 2nd ed.), $9.95.

White, J.A. & Heston, L. (1983). *Dementia: A Practical Guide to Alzheimer's Disease and Related Diseases.* W.B. Freeman & Co.

REFERENCES

Alzheimer's Association (1985, November 15). Understanding and caring for the person with Alzheimer's Disease. *Patient Care,* p. 73.

APA (1987). *Diagnostic and Statistical Manual of Mental Disorders (Third Edition-Revised) DSM-III-R.* Washington, D.C.: American Psychiatric Association.

Bachman, D. L., Wolf, P. A., Linn, R., Knoefel, J. E., Cobb, J., Belanger, A., D'Agostino, R. B., & White, L. R. (1992). Prevalence of dementia and probable senile dementia of the Alzheimer type in the Framingham study. *Neurology,* *42,* 115-119.

Beck, C., Heacock, P., Mercer, S., & Walton, C. (1992). Decreasing caregiver assistance with older adults with dementia. In S. Funk, E. Tornquist, M. Champagne, & R. Wiese (Eds.), *Key aspects of elder care* (pp. 308-319). New York: Springer Publishing Co.

Burns, A. (1992). Psychiatric phenomena in dementia of the Alzheimer type. *International Psychogeriatrics,* *4*(Supp. 1), 43-54.

Calvani, M., & Carta, A. (1991). Clinical issues of cognitive enhancers in Alzheimer Disease. *Alzheimer Disease and Associated Disorders,* *5*(Suppl. 1), S25-S31.

Clarefield, A. M. (1988). The reversible dementias: Do they reverse? *Annals of Internal Medicine,* *109,* 476-486.

Cohen, R. A., & Van Nostrand, J. F. (1992). *Highlights from health data on older Americans: United States, 1992.* National Center for Health Statistics. U.S. Department of Health and Human Services.

Cummings, J., Millet, B., Hill, M. A., & Neshkes, R. (1987). Neuropsychiatric aspects of multi-infarct dementia and dementia of the Alzheimer type. *Archives of Neurology,* *44,* 389-393.

Doty, R. L., Reyes, P. F., & Gregor, T. (1987). Presence of both odor identification and detection deficits in Alzheimer's disease. *Brain Research Bulletin, 18*(5), 597-600.

Evans, D. A., Funkenstein, H. H., Albert, M. S., Scherr, P. A., Cook, N. R., Chown, M. J., Hebert, L. E., Hennekens, C. H., & Taylor, J. O. (1989). Prevalence of Alzheimer's disease in a community population of older persons. *Journal of the American Medical Association, 262*(18), 2551-2556.

Fabiszewski, K. J. (1986). Caring for the Alzheimer's patient. *Gerodontology, 6* (2), 53-58.

Flint, A. J. (1991). Delusions, hallucinations and depression in Alzheimer's disease: a biological perspective. *American Journal of Alzheimers Care and Related Disorders Research, 6*, 21-29.

Forette, F., Henry, J. F., & Orgogozo, J. M. (1989). Reliability of clinical criteria for the diagnosis of dementia: a longitudinal multicenter study. *Archives of Neurology, 46*, 646-648.

Gatz, M., Bengtson, V. L., & Blum, M. J. (1990). Caregiving families. In J. E. Birren & K. W. Schaie (Eds.), *Handbook of the psychology of aging* (pp. 404-426). San Diego: Academic Press.

George, L. K., & Gwyther, L. P. (1986). Caregiver well-being: A multidimensional examination of family caregivers of demented adults. *Gerontologist, 26*(3), 248-252.

Guze, B. H., Hoffman, J. M., Baxter, L. R., Mazziotta, J. C., & Phelps, M. E. (1991). Functional brain imaging and Alzheimer-type dementia. *Alzheimer Disease and Associated Disorders, 5* (4), 215-230.

Gwyther, L. P. (1985). *Care of Alzheimer's Patients: A Manual for Nursing Home Staff*. Chicago: Alzheimer's Association.

Gwyther, L. P. (1991, November 15). General guidelines for caregivers. *Patient Care*, p. 72.

Hall, G. R. (1988). Care of the patient with Alzheimer's disease living at home. *Nursing Clinics of North America, 23* (1), 31- 46.

Harrell, L. E. (1991). Alzheimer's disease. *Southern Medical Journal, 84*(5 Suppl. 1), S32-40.

Jarvik, L. F., Berg, L., Bartus, R., Heston, L., Leith, N., Phelps, C., Shader, R., & Whitehouse, P. (1990). Clinical drug trials in Alzheimer Disease, What are some of the issues? *Alzheimer Disease and Associated Disorders, 4*(4), 193-202.

Jorm, A. F., Fratiglioni, L., & Winblad, B. (1993). Differential diagnosis in dementia. *Archives of Neurology, 50*(1), 72-77.

Jorm, A. F., Korten, A. E., & Henderson, A. S. (1987). The prevalence of dementia: a quantitative integration of the literature. *Acta Psychiatrica Scandia, 76*, 465-479.

Katzman, R., & Jackson, J. E. (1991). Alzheimer disease: basic and clinical advances. *Journal of the American Geriatrics Society, 39*(5), 516-525.

Kent, D. (1992). Creating a home that speaks their language. *Aging*. U.S. Department of Health and Human Services, Numbers 363-364, pp. 32-34.

Khatchaturian, Z. (1987). Status of Alzheimer's disease research. In H. J. Altman (Eds.), *Alzheimer's disease: problems, prospects, and perspectives* (pp. 183-189). New York: Plenum Press.

Kramer, S. I., & Reifler, B. V. (1992). Depression, dementia, and reversible dementia. *Clinics in Geriatric Medicine, 8*(2), 288-97.

Lowenthal, D. T., & Nadeau, S. E. (1991). Drug-induced dementia. *Southern Medical Journal, 84* (5, Suppl. 1), S24-31.

McKhann, G., Drachman, D., Folstein, M., Katzman, R., Price, D., & Stadlan, E. M. (1984). Clinical diagnosis of Alzheimer's disease: Report of the NINCDS-ADRDA work group under the auspices of Department of Health and Human Services Task Force on Alzheimer's Disease. *Neurology, 34*(7), 939-944.

Morris, J. C., Heyman, A., Mohs, R. C., Hughes, J., Van Belle, G., Fillenbaum, G., Mellits, E. D., & Clark, C. (1989). The Consortium to Establish a Registry for Alzheimer's Disease (CERAD). Part I. Clinical and neuropsychological assessment of Alzheimer's disease. *Neurology, 39*, 1159-1165.

Morris, J. C., & Rubin, E. H. (1991). Clinical diagnosis and course of Alzheimer's disease. *The Psychiatric Clinics of North America, 14*(2), 223-235.

Mortimer, J. A., Van Duijn, C. M., Chandra V. et al. (1991). Head trauma as a risk factor for Alzheimer's disease: A collaborative re-analysis of case-control studies. *International Journal of Epidemiology, 20*, S28-S35.

NIA (1992). *Progress report on Alzheimer's disease.* U.S. Department of Health and Human Services (NIH Publication No. 92-3409).

Nussbaum, M., Treves, T. A., & Korczyn, A. D. (1992). DSM-III criteria for primary degenerative dementia and multi-infarct dementia. *Alzheimer Disease and Associated Disorders, 6*(2), 111-118.

Rabins, P. V. (1992). Prevention of mental disorder in the elderly: Current perspectives and future prospects. *Journal of the American Geriatrics Society, 40*, 727-733.

Rabins, P., Mace, M., & Lucas, M. (1982). The impact of dementia on the family. *Journal of the American Medical Association, 248*, 333-335.

Reisberg, B. (Ed.). (1983). *Alzheimer's disease: The standard reference.* New York: The Free Press.

Rezek, D. L. (1987). Olfactory deficits as a neurologic sign in dementia of the Alzheimer type. *Archives of Neurology, 44*, 1030-1032.

Ritchie, K., & Touchon, J. (1992). Heterogeneity in senile dementia of the Alzheimer type: Individual differences, progressive deterioration or clinical subtypes? *Journal of Clinical Epidemiology, 45*(12), 1391-1398.

Schoenberg, B. S., Kokmen, E., & Okazaki, H. (1987). Alzheimer's disease and other dementing illnesses in a defined United States population: Incidence rates and clinical features. *Annals of Neurology, 22*, 724-729.

Somerfield, M. R., Weisman, C. S., Ury, W., Chase, G. A., & Folstein, M. F. (1991). Physician practices in the diagnosis of dementing disorders. *Journal of the American Geriatrics Society, 39*(2), 172-175.

Souder, E. (1992). The consumer approach to recruitment of elderly subjects. *Nursing Research, 41* (5), 314-316.

St. George-Hyslop, P. H., Haines, J. L., Farrer, L. A., Polinsky, R., Van Broeckhoven, C., Goate, A., & McLachlan, D. R. (1990). Genetic linkage studies suggest that Alzheimer's disease is not a single homogeneous disorder. *Nature,*
347, 194-197.

Tackenberg, J. (1992). Teaching caregivers about Alzheimer's disease. *Nursing*
92, 22(5), 75-78.

Teri, L., Rabins, P., Whitehouse, P., Berg, L., Reisberg, B., Sunderland, T., Eichel-
man, B., & Phelps, C. (1992). Management of behavior disturbance in Alzheimer disease: Current knowledge and future directions. *Alzheimer Disease*
and Associated Disorders, 6(2), 77-88.

Van Ort, S., & Phillips, L. (1992). Feeding nursing home residents with Alzheimer's disease. *Geriatric Nursing, 13* (5), 249-253.

Weiner, M. F. (1991). *The dementias: diagnosis and management.* Washington,
D.C.: American Psychiatric Press.

Weiner, M. F., Bruhn, M., Svetlik, D., Tintner, R., & Hom, J. (1991). Experiences
with depression in a dementia clinic. *Journal of Clinical Psychiatry, 52* (5),
234-238.

Wells, C. E. (1985). Organic syndromes: dementia. In H. I. Kaplan & B. J. Sadock
(Eds.), *Comprehensive Textbook of Psychiatry.* Baltimore: Williams & Wilkins.

Whitehouse, P. J. (1991). Treatment of Alzheimer disease. *Alzheimer Disease and*
Associated Disorders, 5(Suppl. 1), S32-S36.

Wiseman, E. J. (in press). Psychiatric Disorders of Late Life: Drug and Alcohol
Abuse. In H. I. Kaplan & B. J. Sadock (Eds.), *Comprehensive Textbook of*
Psychiatry. Baltimore: Williams & Wilkins.

Living Productively with Sensory Loss

Cheryl H. Kinderknecht, ACSW, LMSW
J. Dianne Garner, DSW

SUMMARY. As the avenues for fully perceiving and experiencing life, our sensory organs are the bridge between Self and the outside world. Of the many disorders affecting the senses of the older woman, those that affect vision and hearing have the greatest potential for disrupting her activities of daily living, and diminishing her quality of life and level of independence. While adapting to and coping successfully with sensory loss may require significant effort and adjustment on the part of the afflicted older woman, strategies designed to maximize the older woman's function, her sense of personal control, and her social support system can mediate the negative effects of the sensory loss.

Often simply taken for granted, the five senses: sight, hearing, taste, smell and touch are our avenues for fully perceiving and experiencing life. Constantly supplying our brains with sensory input, the five senses allow us to be interacters with and receptors of the world about us. In short, our sensory organs are the bridge between the Self and the outside world. While the term 'sensory loss' is essentially self-explanatory, it covers a continuum ranging from minor, inconsequential sensory diminishment to total and dev-

---

Cheryl H. Kinderknecht is Administrative Officer, Behavioral Sciences Regulatory Board, Topeka, KS.

J. Dianne Garner is Professor and Chair, Department of Social Work at Washburn University, Topeka, KS.

[Haworth co-indexing entry note]: "Living Productively with Sensory Loss." Kinderknecht, Cheryl H., and J. Dianne Garner. Co-published simultaneously in the *Journal of Women & Aging* (The Haworth Press, Inc.) Vol. 5, No. 3/4, 1993, pp. 155-180; and: *Women and Healthy Aging: Living Productively in Spite of It All* (ed: J. Dianne Garner, and Alice A. Young), The Haworth Press, Inc., 1993, pp. 155-180. Multiple copies of this article/chapter may be purchased from The Haworth Document Delivery Center [1-800-3-HAWORTH; 9:00 a.m.-5:00 p.m. (EST)].

astating loss of function. Whether due to processes of aging, under-lying disease or a combination of both, the partial or full loss of any sensory function has significant implications for the older woman. Her independence and her quality of life may be markedly curtailed by severe or multiple sensory losses.

While the rate of progression is variable, certain age-related changes in sensory function can be a normal part of the aging process. Age-related changes in the structure and function of the eye may result in the loss of fine vision, poor night vision, higher sensitivity to glare, diminished peripheral vision and the need for greater background contrasts. Beyond the age of 50, changes in hearing result in a decrease in ability to hear certain sounds or tones or to distinguish between words with similar sounds. Chemosensory disorders involving taste and smell are not uncommon over the age of 60. The ability to smell declines more rapidly in men than women and can contribute to decreased taste as well (National Institute on Aging [NIoA], 1987). The number and size of the taste buds diminishes, resulting in a less distinct discrimination between the four basic tastes of sweet, sour, bitter and salt (Pearson & Beck, 1989). Other factors impinging upon the senses of taste and smell include nasal obstructions, allergies, upper dentures that obstruct the palate and the side-effects of prescription and/or over-the-counter medications (Pearson & Beck, 1989).

Age and disease-related processes may also interfere with mus-culoskeletal, neurosensory and circulatory function, resulting in an altered or absent sense of touch. Symptoms include numbness, tingling, diminished or absent tactile sensation and diminished or absent sensation of heat, cold and pain in the affected body part(s). For many women, the processes of aging are accompanied by subtle and very gradual changes in sensory functioning. For others, the presence of disease or physiological disorders further diminishes or totally obliterates her sensory functioning.

Of the many disorders affecting the senses of aging women, "those that affect vision and hearing have the greatest potential for disabling physical and emotional impact" (Pearson & Beck, 1989, p. 167). Because of their centrality among the sensory processes and their impairing predominance among the aged, the focus here is on vision and hearing loss. Incidence, major causes and consequences of age-related vision and hearing loss are presented, along with treatment options and issues. Finally, strategies for enhancing the capacity for productive living are discussed. Given the demographics on longevity, statistics concerning "the elderly" as a group are believed to disproportionately pertain to older women unless otherwise stipulated.

PREVALENCE OF OCCURRENCE AND RISK FACTORS

Visual impairment is the second most prevalent physical impairment among persons age 65 and older (National Center for Health Statistics [NCHS], 1982). The elderly as a group, particularly the oldest old, are more susceptible to vision loss than younger people since the incidence of vision impairment increases dramatically with age (NCHS, 1982). Half of this country's visually impaired citizens are 65 or older, and older individuals account for one-third of all visits for medical eye care (United States Senate Special Committee on Aging [USSCA], 1991). The majority of people with visual problems in late life are women (Kirchner & Lowman, 1978) and most newly impaired women are poor, have concurrent health conditions and are unrecognized as impaired when they have some remaining vision (Wineburg, 1984). Elderly women who are newly visually impaired or blinded may have difficulty with adaptive demands because of overlapping physiological problems.

Typically, vision loss is but one of several coexisting disabilities among the elderly cohort (Branch, Horowitz, & Carr, 1989). At least two-thirds of the visually impaired elderly experience concurrent health conditions or impairments (Kirchner, 1985). Diminished or absent vision dramatically increases the likelihood of falls, the most common cause of fatal injury in older persons (NIA, 1988). Visually impaired elderly also tend to have more physical ailments and experience more fluctuations in appetite than do their non-affected counterparts (Grieg, West, & Overbury, 1986). The number of older people with severe visual impairments more than doubled between 1960 and 1990, leaping from 1.25 million to 2.6 million (Alliance for Aging Research [AAR], 1992). With the baby boom generation coming to retirement age, it is projected that by year

2030 there will be nearly six million severely visually impaired individuals nationwide the vast majority of whom will be women.

The four leading causes of vision loss among the elderly are macular degeneration, cataracts, glaucoma and diabetic retinopathy (AAR, 1992). It is estimated that among the over 65 age cohort, 3% suffer from glaucoma, 11% from macular degeneration and as many as two-thirds have some form of lens opacity (NIoA, 1985). Age-related macular degeneration (AMD) is the leading cause of blindness in Americans age 65 and older (AAR, 1992). Of the nearly 34 million Americans who will be 65 and older in 1995, it is estimated that 1.7 will have decreased vision secondary to AMD. While glaucoma can occur at any age, it is more prevalent among the cohort age 40 years old and over (Pearson & Beck, 1989). The second leading cause of blindness among all Americans, glaucoma is the leading cause of blindness among African Americans (USSSCA, 1991). Among American adults ages forty-one to sixty, diabetic retinopathy is at present the leading cause of blindness (Barlow, Siegal, Edwards, & Doress, 1987). Almost half of the diabetics who become blind are over age 65 (USSSCA, 1991).

In 1987, the number of people of all ages in the United States with a hearing impairment was estimated to be 20,994,000, or 1 in 10, of whom 350,000 are profoundly deaf (Schoenborn & Marano, 1988). About 10 million of these individuals, or nearly half of the hearing impaired population, are age 65 or older (AAR, 1992). Many of these individuals over age 65 are affected by presbycusis (NIoA, 1983), a gradual age-related decline in hearing acuity that interferes with speech perception (USSSCA, 1991). Currently, approximately 30 percent of adults age 65 through 74 and about 50 percent of those age 75 through 79 suffer some degree of hearing loss.

Among the elderly, the presence of a hearing impairment is often associated with a higher incidence of ambulation difficulties and balance problems, resulting in an increased likelihood of falls. Bess et al. (1989) found that among the elderly hearing and communication dysfunction are associated with global dysfunction: specifically, the degree of overall functional impairment increases in relationship to the degree of hearing impairment. When allowed to progress, hearing loss diminishes quality of life and constitutes a threat to safety due to inability to hear alarms and other signals warning of danger (Pearson & Beck, 1989).

Demographically, hearing loss is more prevalent among males than among females; males constitute 60% of those with hearing loss (Better Hearing Institute [BHI]). In addition to gender differences, hearing impairment is proportionately overrepresented among whites, persons in households earning less than $7,000 annually and those with less than 12 years of education (Ries, 1985). By the year 2050, 26 million individuals are expected to have a hearing impairment.

PHYSIOLOGICAL IMPACTS
AND PSYCHOSOCIAL IMPLICATIONS

Knowing the prevalence of and risk factors for visual and hearing impairments is an important consideration for professionals who serve the elderly. However, it is critical to go beyond the surface of demographics. Behind the figures and facts are the women whose lives may change as a result of loss of vision or hearing. Personal care, grooming, dressing, cooking, eating, ambulation, management of household, shopping, banking and conducting business matters are routine, elementary affairs of daily living for the sighted. To the visually impaired, these skills are obstacles to independence unless specifically mastered. Moreover, because of the ambiguity of their poorly defined role within a sighted world, low vision women may have difficulty maintaining their pre-existing social roles.

As a group, hearing impaired people are isolated from the general population. Despite the use of hearing aids and other assistance, the impaired individual may struggle to hear, feel out of place in conversation and frequently miss the intended meaning of the message communicated (Beck, 1989). In an attempt to minimize the disruption of their everyday lives, some may be inclined to camouflage their impairment by pretending to hear and understand. Embarrassment or fear may reduce the likelihood of asking for repetition or clarification. The end result is that the hearing impaired woman often remains on the periphery of communication, as an observer rather than a participant. Common leisure activities such as listening to the radio, watching and making sense of television or films, having a casual conversation and visiting on the telephone are often frustrating or impossible for the hearing impaired. Boredom and loss of self-esteem are also serious problems (Pearson & Beck, 1989). The elderly woman's reaction to hearing impairment and its accompanying frustrations may include embarrassment, withdrawal, social isolation, fear and depression.

Sensory loss often concurrently involves a variety of psychological and social changes. With the onset of age-related sensory loss, changes occur in customary roles, relationships and routines. Previously enjoyed sources of interaction, entertainment and leisure may no longer be pleasurable or possible. The onset of age-related sensory loss often coincides closely with retirement, making the transition to retirement more stressful. The older woman must cope with sensory loss at the same time she experiences income reduction and the loss of workplace social roles and social supports. In addition, widowhood, with all its accompanying losses, may occur at the approximate time age-related sensory losses are manifesting themselves.

Older women affected by sensory impairment may experience a range of psychological reactions which include grief, confusion, anger, fear, depression, loss of control and loss of self-esteem. Unresolved, these psychological responses may constrict the individual's daily activities, interests and physical capacities. Psychological components of new sensory loss may include feelings of vulnerability, insecurity and self-doubt. Multiple factors may contribute to this phenomenon, including the woman's physical and psychological dependency, social isolation and diminished opportunities for normative experiences and the often over-protective attitudes of family, friends, health care providers and society.

As opposed to a gradual age-related sensory loss, the abrupt or traumatic loss of vision or hearing may involve a dramatic change in the woman's self-identity and functioning. Abruptness and extent of the loss can have devastating consequences on her customary roles, relationships, activities of daily living, employment and economic security. Acute grief reactions can be expected, as can disruptions in body image.

Feelings of fear, frustration and hopelessness associated with sensory loss may lead to maladaptive coping mechanisms such as denial, depression, isolation and learned helplessness. How the individual defines her loss and the meaning ascribed to it determines adaptive and adjustment capacity. Factors that influence the visually or hearing impaired woman's adjustment may include age at onset, degree and stability of residual function, pre-existing personality characteristics, coping style and her support network. Since much of the adjusting and adapting process requires creativity and problem-solving abilities, intelligence and common sense also impact upon her options and outcomes. Reactions of significant others strongly influence the ultimate psychosocial impacts of sensory loss. Family acceptance is closely linked to the older woman's personal adjustment. Individual self-worth can be jeopardized when significant others over-protect, patronize or fail to provide her with opportunities for interactive behaviors.

PROCESSES OF AGING AND CAUSES OF VISUAL AND HEARING IMPAIRMENT

Visual Impairment

Certain changes in the structure and function of the eye are normal variations associated with the process of aging. While some of these age-related changes may interfere with vision, vision loss is not an inevitable result of aging (AAR, 1992).

Presbyopia, sometimes called 'old age vision,' is the most common age-related visual change (Pearson & Beck, 1989). At about 40, changes to the structure of the eye include a reduction in the elasticity of the lens and the muscles that control it. The inability to focus clearly on near objects necessitates the use of magnification for reading and work requiring fine vision. The pupil of the eye becomes smaller and sometimes irregular in shape, reducing the speed and the efficiency of the eye's reactivity to light changes. The aging eye then requires more illumination to be able to see (Pearson & Beck, 1989). To have good visual acuity at age 60, one needs twice the light needed at age 20; by age 80, three times the light is needed to see objects well (Ebersole & Hess, 1981; NIoA, 1987).

The criteria for legal blindness is visual acuity of 20/200 or worse in the better eye after maximum correction, or visual fields constricted to 20 degrees or less. This means that even with the best possible correction the person has no more than 10% of the normal vision in the better eye (Braille Institute, n.d.). The broader category of severe visual impairment is defined as the inability, despite the best correction, to read regular newspaper print (Branch, Horowitz, & Carr, 1989). A diverse variety of eye diseases and injuries can contribute to visual impairment or blindness.

Age-related macular degeneration involves atrophy or damage of the macular disc, resulting in loss of central visual acuity (NIoA, 1987). The macula, the part of the retina that controls the acuity or sharpness of central vision, gradually ceases to function, possibly related to decreased blood supply (Pearson & Beck, 1989). This painless disease generally occurs bilaterally and results in symptoms of darkened or distorted vision and loss of color vision. Cataracts involve an opacity, partial or complete, of one or both eyes, resulting in a progressive loss of vision. The degree of loss depends on the location, size and density of the opacity. Cataracts can be caused by injury, radiation exposure, infections or inflammation of the eye (Barlow et al., 1987). Most commonly, cataracts occur later in life as a result of degenerative changes in the lens of the eye. Characterized by a gradual increase in pressure within the eye (interocular pressure) resulting from the inadequate drainage of fluid, glaucoma slowly causes progressive loss of peripheral vision. Uncontrolled, glaucoma causes loss of central vision and ultimately results in blindness. Symptoms may include eye pain, nausea, headaches, seeing colored halos around lights and decreased visual sharpness. Diabetic retinopathy, a major cause of vision loss or blindness in diabetics, involves the gradual deterioration of the retina due to diabetes-related eye problems such as capillary hemorrhage, retinal exudates, scarring and swelling. Similar retinal damage occurs in association with untreated or uncontrolled hypertension.

Another eye disease resulting in age-related visual impairment or blindness is optic nerve atrophy. Optic nerve atrophy is generally caused by persistent intraocular pressure, chronic inflammation or other conditions that damage the optic nerve. Visual loss is proportional to the degree of nerve atrophy. When optic nerve pressure is associated with an underlying condition, the timely treatment of the underlying condition may result in improvement or elimination of visual impairment. If the underlying condition remains undetected or untreated, permanent and irreversible damage to or atrophy of the optic nerve may result. Other conditions or diseases can contribute to vision loss or blindness among the elderly, including cerebrovascular accidents (strokes), target-organ damage to the retina associated with untreated or poorly controlled hypertension, cancer that involves the eye or certain parts of the brain, eye infections and trauma.

Hearing Impairment

As sound passes through the ear, it sets off a chain reaction. Components of the ear sense, amplify, relay and transmit the information to the brain. Sound vibrations are collected by the outer ear and funneled through the ear canal to the eardrum. The bones of the middle ear amplify the vibrations, causing fluid in the inner ear to vibrate and stimulate the tiny nerve endings called hair cells. The hair cells transform the vibrations into electrical impulses which travel to the brain. Vibratory differences picked up by each of our two ears create a stereophonic effect which helps the brain locate and identify the origin of the sound. There are two major types of hearing loss: sensorineural and conductive. When components of both sensorineural and conductive impairment are present, it is referred to as a 'mixed' hearing loss. A third type of hearing loss, which rarely occurs, is referred to as central deafness.

The predominant type of hearing impairment, sensorineural or 'nerve' hearing loss, is caused by problems in the inner ear as a result of damage to or destruction of the hair cells and/or nerve fibers in the inner ear. The most common causes of sensorineural hearing loss are the aging processes, prolonged exposure to loud levels of noise or exposure to a sudden, extremely high decibel noise. Other causes include high fever, medication effects, improper diet or predisposing genetic factors.

As they age, many individuals experience gradual and progressive sensorineural hearing loss, resulting in reduced hearing acuity (USSSCA, 1991). The most common age-related sensorineural hearing loss is presbycusis which generally affects individuals, particularly men, over the age of 50. Age-related changes associated with presbycusis usually do not lead to total deafness. The result of presbycusis is a loss of hearing acuity, including the inability to hear high-pitched sounds, difficulty distinguishing common consonants and inability to discriminate speech that is rapid or is occurring in environments with background noises (Pearson & Beck, 1989). Symptoms of presbycusis are different in each person, suggesting that genetic predisposition and neurochemical faults may be superimposed with normal age-related changes and repeated lifelong exposure to noise (USSSC, 1991). Age-related hearing losses associated with presbycusis can be accompanied by hearing problems caused by other factors such as vascular changes, tumors, effects of certain drugs on hearing, disease or the environment (Pearson & Beck, 1989).

Conductive hearing loss involves the inability of the outer or middle ear to conduct sound waves to the inner ear. Usually this is due to an obstruction in some part of the ear that impedes or eliminates the transmission of physical vibrations through air, bone or tissue. Conductive hearing loss may be caused by conditions such as excessive cerumen (ear wax), infection, a punctured eardrum or the congenital or traumatic immobilization of the bones of the middle ear.

Caused by the damage to the nerve centers to the brain, central deafness involves the inability to understand language even though the ability to perceive sound levels is not affected. The causes may include extended illnesses with a high fever, head injury, vascular problems or tumors. Other otologic conditions common to the elderly include tinnitus and Meniere's disease. While not a cause of hearing loss, tinnitus and other otological symptoms such as inner ear pressure, unsteadiness and dizziness associated with Meniere's disease often accompany decreased hearing. Commonly referred to as ringing in the ears, tinnitus is the perception of sound in the absence of an acoustic stimulus. Tinnitus may involve buzzing, ringing, roaring, clicking, whistling or hissing. It may be intermittent, continuous or pulsatile (synchronous with the heartbeat). The causes of tinnitus include wax buildup, perforation of the eardrum, fluid accumulation behind the eardrum, local or systemic infectious processes, allergy, injury or toxicity. Tinnitus may also be the signal of an underlying condition, such as cardiovascular disease, anemia, hypothyroidism or certain neoplasms. Medical investigation is warranted so that treatment focuses on alleviating the underlying cause, rather than simply masking the symptoms. A disorder of the inner ear, Meniere's disease is characterized by recurrent debilitating vertigo associated with nausea and vomiting, sensory hearing loss and tinnitus. The etiology of Meniere's disease is unknown, and the frequency and severity of attacks may vary.

MEDICAL TREATMENT OPTIONS AND ISSUES

Since several types of disease-related causes of vision impairment can be avoided or their functional consequences dramatically reduced, early detection, diagnosis and treatment of age-related conditions is indicated. To prevent accidental, traumatic eye injuries, the use of protective eyewear is recommended. Similarly, the early identification of hearing impairment and hearing conservation methods offer the best 'preventive medicine.' Women who are regularly exposed to high noise levels should have a hearing test at least once a year, and every woman suspected of having a hearing loss should have her hearing tested, especially older women. Any noise loud enough to prohibit normal levels of conversation can cause hearing loss, particularly after repeated or prolonged exposure. Wearing hearing protection in noisy environments can protect and preserve hearing acuity. Because some medications affect hearing, it is also pertinent to have a physician outline the potential side-effects of any prescribed drugs so that ototoxic drugs can be avoided if possible (BHI, 1989).

While primary prevention is a critical consideration for the preservation of sight and hearing, it is realistic to acknowledge that increased longevity and genetic factors will ultimately impact on sensory functioning. Despite the best prevention efforts, there is the likelihood that treatment might be needed at some point during the later years.

Visual Impairment

Bifocal glasses or lenses are routinely and effectively used to compensate for structural and functional change in vision associated with presbyopia. With this simple correction, visual tasks such as reading and sewing are again possible without strain. Medical treatment for macular degeneration is presently limited, but some success has been reported with the use of laser therapy to slow or halt the course of the disease (Pearson & Beck, 1989). Currently, a variety of research investigations related to AMD are underway. Some of these investigations include: genetic research into inherited diseases of the retina; the efficacy of nutritional supplements in preventing or slowing the progression of AMD; and advanced research into transplantation of cells in the retina (AAR, 1992).

Not all cataracts need to be removed. The factor influencing surgical intervention is the degree to which the cataract interferes with vision. In those cases where medical intervention is indicated, the standard treatments associated with cataracts are the surgical extraction of the opaque lens, with replacement of an artificial plastic lens in the eye or the use of special contact lens or eyeglasses. In 90 to 95% of cataract extractions, the surgery restores vision that allows patients to return to their usual activities of daily living (Luckman & Sorenson, 1987). While the implanted lenses or the extended-wear contact lenses generally restore a full field of vision, there may be some distortion with the cataract eyeglasses (Barlow et al., 1987).

Glaucoma treatment first involved medication therapy, in the form of eyedrops, to improve fluid drainage or to slow fluid formation. If eyedrops were unsuccessful in bringing the intraocular pressure to an acceptable level, the physician used laser surgery to create a tiny hole in the coat of the eye or stretch open holes in the drainage tissue. Recent studies indicate that intraocular pressure can be better controlled through medication therapy when laser surgery has been used as the initial component of treatment (USSSCA 1991). It is a myth that glaucoma inevitably leads to blindness: with early detection and prompt treatment, glaucoma can usually be controlled and blindness prevented.

Diabetic retinopathy was uncommon until a few decades ago: improved diabetic survival rates mean that now many diabetics live to suffer the complications of the disease (Barlow et al., 1987). Laser surgery to coagulate hemorrhaging retinal capillaries is a useful and effective treatment in the early stages of diabetic or hypertensive retinopathy. Good control of the underlying disease is considered an essential component of treatment as well. Early diagnosis increases the likelihood of controlling this disease of the retina's blood vessels and eye fluid (Barlow et al., 1987).

When trauma severely damages the eyeball or severs the eye muscles or optic nerve, enucleation (surgical removal of the eye) may be necessary. Enucleation may also be necessary for ocular cancers or with severe, persistent, and painful eye infections. In such cases, an eye patch or a prosthetic eye is utilized for cosmetic purposes.

Hearing Impairment

With recent medical and technological advances, it is now possible to perform comprehensive testing to determine if hearing loss exists, the extent and nature of the loss and the benefits possible through treatment. Special auditory tests identify the exact location of the auditory impairment and allow objective, complete identification of middle ear and nerve function disorders. One such test, auditory brainstem response (ABR) testing, provides medical diagnosis of auditory disorders in difficult-to-test patients and populations such as the elderly with cognitive or multiple disabilities.

Since many causes of hearing loss can be remediated through medical or surgical means, an evaluation by a physician is necessary to determine the cause of, and the pathology associated with, the hearing loss. This should occur before the patient is seen by a hearing aid specialist. Hearing aid specialists are required by the Food and Drug Administration (FDA) to advise a client to consult promptly with a licensed physician when there is visible congenital or traumatic deformity of the ear, a history of acute or chronic dizziness, visible evidence of cerumen accumulation or a foreign body in the ear and pain or discomfort of the ear. This is also the case when there is a history of active drainage from the ear or a sudden or rapidly progressive hearing loss within the previous 90 days (National Hearing Aid Society [NHAS], 1988).

Many conductive hearing impairments can be successfully treated by medical or surgical measures. Simple flushing can eliminate the buildup of cerumen in the ear canal, and fluid buildup behind the eardrum is often responsive to antibiotics. In some cases, surgical drainage of the fluid through an incision in the eardrum is necessary, and a pressure equalizing tube is inserted to prevent further problems. Fixation of the hearing bones (otosclerosis) can be corrected through a surgical procedure called a stapedectomy. The profoundly deaf or those whose residual hearing is severely limited may be helped by use of a cochlear implant. Hearing aids are also of considerable assistance for conductive hearing loss.

Although sensorineural hearing loss may not be correctable through surgery or medication, a hearing aid may sharpen hearing acuity when there is sufficient residual hearing present. While it offsets the hearing loss, the aid will not restore hearing to normal. When sensorineural hearing loss is secondary to medication side-effects, removing the ototoxic drug generally restores hearing acuity. For example, large dosages of aspirin may be prescribed for arthritis or other musculoskeletal conditions, resulting in a temporary hearing loss. Switching to a non-aspirin product will often remedy the hearing problem (Barlow, Doress, & Siegal, 1987).

With tinnitus, when the symptoms are pronounced, those with normal hearing may be helped by a tinnitus masking device worn like a hearing aid. For those with both tinnitus and a hearing loss, a hearing aid may drown out the ringing with other ambient noise. A definitive treatment of Meniere's disease is still elusive. Some patients may benefit from otological surgery, while symptomatic relief of the vertigo and feelings of inner ear pressure is achieved through medication. Central deafness cannot be treated medically or surgically, although some patients benefit from special training by an audiologist or speech therapist.

Because many causes of hearing loss can now be resolved or lessened through medical or surgical means, patients should be encouraged to seek preliminary medical evaluation, prior to being fitted for hearing aids. This ensures that correctable otological problems are eliminated or reduced, and if a hearing aid will be beneficial, it is suited to the type and extent of the patient's hearing loss. With monaural fitting, a single aid is used for the best ear, while binaural fitting involves aids for both ears. The latter approach provides stereophonic hearing, allowing the hearer to localize the source of sound, as is the case with normal hearing. There is no single hearing instrument that is suitable in all cases; the correct device depends on the type and nature of the hearing impairment. There are four basic types of hearing aids: the in-the-ear (ITE) device; the behind-the-ear (BTE) model; the eyeglass aid; and, the body aid. The ITE, BTE and eyeglass aid are all generally effective for mild to severe hearing loss. Both sensorineural and bone conduction hearing aids are available in the eyeglass model. The body aid is generally used for severe to profound hearing loss and is considered more suitable for use by children (NHAS, 1988).

Rehabilitation is an often overlooked treatment option when vision or hearing impairment is present. Unfortunately, rehabilitation services have historically been targeted to children, young adults and middle-aged adults. A philosophy of vocational rehabilitation prevails, prioritizing those with employment potential for rehabilitation services. Although changing, the prevailing attitudes may still exclude the elderly, particularly the old-old, forcing them to adapt and cope with a host of unmet needs, and increasing their risks for functional dependence and/or institutionalization. In addition to constituting a viable treatment option for the older woman, rehabilitation also represents a potent strategy for living productively with a vision or a hearing loss.

STRATEGIES FOR PRODUCTIVE AGING: MAKING THE MOST OUT OF LESS

The older woman faced with a significant sensory loss is challenged to compensate for the loss by making both subtle and radical changes in her activities and her environment. Variable by the degree of individual impairment, sensory loss may precipitate the need for adopting new routines as well as adapting the old in order to continue experiencing and enjoying life to the maximum degree.

Certain strategies are useful for maximizing residual functioning, allowing the older woman to make the most out of less as she strives to continue to live her life and adapt to the processes of aging in a productive manner. Regardless of the degree of impairment, strategies for living and aging productively should include psychosocial elements as well as physiological and practical considerations. Useful approaches toward continued productive living and aging include the following: environmental adaptation and practical considerations; rehabilitation; adaptive devices and concrete resources; enhancing the woman's sense of personal control; and the development or maintenance of an active social support system.

Environmental Adaptation and Practical Considerations

With either vision or hearing impairment, practical adaptations in the environment can enhance quality of life by maximizing residual function and safety. Practical considerations for family members and care providers are also essential ingredients in maximizing the older woman's residual functioning and psychosocial adjustment.

For the visually impaired, adequate direct lighting should be available for reading and close work. Glare from lights, windows and mirrors should be avoided to reduce distortions in visual acuity and depth perception. Bright colors such as yellows, oranges and reds are more visible and provide improved contrast differentiation from background colors. If the residual vision prohibits reading printed material, a 'reader' will be required on a regular basis to assist with mail and business matters.

Safety in ambulation is an important consideration for the older woman with a visual impairment. Tips for enhancing safety include keeping the 'foot traffic' pathways and hallways free of clutter, removing or tacking down loose scatter rugs, installing handrails, painting contrast marking at step edges and ensuring adequate, indirect lighting for all interior and exterior stairwells. When ambulation assistance is needed, the older woman should take the arm of the assisting individual. Walking a half-step behind, she will be able to 'sense' and anticipate direction, steps or curbs. The assistant's relevant and timely verbal cues relating to distance and changes in direction or gradation further allow the older woman to mentally plan the route to be navigated. Such cues also provide a measure of predictability and personal control.

If the older woman is severely visually impaired, special considerations should be employed when she is ambulating in an unfamiliar environment. Furniture placement and any obstacles to mobility should be described. When being seated, guide her hand to the chair and alert her if the seat happens to be higher or lower than that of a standard chair. If the older woman will be dining or handling materials from a table or desk, place objects within her immediate reach and describe their placement as on a clock face: for instance, cup at 9 o'clock.

Reducing or eliminating background noise is an important consideration for maximizing the residual hearing of the impaired older woman. Strategically placed seating which favors her better ear minimizes auditory distortion. Good lighting assists in more effective lip reading and allows her to see the facial features or hand gestures of the speaker, facilitating perception of the speaker's message. In communicating with the older woman with a hearing impairment, others should position themselves near good light so lip movements, facial expressions and gestures can be clearly seen. Others' position and distance should be guided by what is most effective for the older woman. Speech volume should be slightly louder than normal, but shouting does not make the message any clearer and sometimes distorts it. The woman should be asked if she can hear clearly and she should have both verbal and nonverbal permission to request repetition. If multiple people are taking part in a conversation, all should be visible and positioned no more than 6 feet from the hearing impaired older woman.

Safety factors for hearing impaired women are best addressed through the use of adaptive amplification devices. Health care and human service providers should bear in mind that those with mild to moderate hearing impairments may be inclined to camouflage the loss from others. Unidentified, hearing loss may cause older women to be wrongly labeled as confused, unresponsive or uncooperative. It is important for professionals to be aware of signs and symptoms that may suggest a hearing impairment. For instance, the hearing impaired may 'favor' their better ear, turning their head slightly to one side, or they may intently watch the speaker's lips and facial expressions. The professional's awareness of the hearing impairment ensures that appropriate practice and treatment considerations are implemented and that referrals for further evaluation, specialized treatment and rehabilitation are made. Overlooking the older woman's hearing impairment can have deleterious effects upon her health, education, understanding, compliance and safety.

Rehabilitation

Rehabilitation represents a particularly potent strategy for productive living. The functional extent or severity of the sensory loss to a large degree dictates the nature and extent of the patient's need for specialized rehabilitation. The degree of rehabilitative need depends heavily upon the amount of residual sensory capacity, the individual's adaptive and coping abilities and the presence or absence of other functional impairments. Rehabilitative capacity and outcome may be impeded when cognitive, physical or concurrent sensory limitations are present.

Rehabilitation treatment associated with vision loss or blindness is geared toward maximizing functional independence. Individuals are trained to use any residual vision functioning effectively, often by relying on special aids (Wineburg, 1984). Rehabilitation training in orientation and mobility enables the visually impaired older woman to move about safely, efficiently and with confidence, making efficient use of her remaining senses. Other rehabilitation training components involve adaptive skill enhancement related to independent living, home management, cooking, personal care management and communication. Training in communication skills may include learning to read and write Braille, or to use special magnification tools, modified typewriters and computers or other sensory aids. Rehabilitation should include educational and recreational activities to assist acceptance of and adaptation to the vision loss, as well as providing opportunities for socialization and life enrichment.

Low vision training programs may be conducted in a training center, in the individual's home or both. Women residing in large, urban areas have more diversified and comprehensive low vision rehabilitation options available, but the needs of the non-urban visually impaired should not be neglected. Short-term residential treatment away from home may be necessary, and it should be borne in mind that non-specialized rehabilitation centers and home health care nurses, physical therapists and occupational therapists can provide beneficial low-vision training.

Regardless of the etiology of the hearing loss, auditory rehabilitation is available for the hearing impaired. Physiological factors that impact upon the severity of the impairment include the patient's age at onset, the severity and rapidity of hearing loss and the degree of residual hearing present. When the degree of hearing impairment is pronounced, alternate communication skills may need to be developed.

Rehabilitation services may include sign language instruction; individually tailored and computerized training in speechreading (lip reading); auditory training, counseling and assistance in everyday listening through custom-designed personal hearing aids. Other rehabilitative services include assistance in specific listening situations (telephone communication, television, group listening situations) through the use of assistive listening devices; cochlear implants, tactile aids and alerting devices for the profoundly deaf; and, counseling and the use of tinnitus maskers for those who suffer ear noises (BHI, 1989). Rehabilitation should address the psychosocial as well as the functional needs of the hearing impaired. Special emphasis should be placed on action-oriented strategies that provide the individual with opportunities for success within her customary environment and activities of daily living. Unfortunately, the majority of adults who are hearing impaired receive inadequate rehabilitation services (Commission on Education of the Deaf, 1988).

Since they are the predominant source of referrals for rehabilitation services, health care and human service providers serve as gatekeepers to the rehabilitation process. When we, as professionals, fail to recognize the rehabilitative needs and potentials of elderly women, we rob them of their potential for maximum functioning, independence and quality of life.

Adaptive Devices and Concrete Resources

Adaptive devices and equipment can dramatically enhance functional capacity, independence and quality of life of the older woman with a sensory impairment. Aids for the visually impaired include magnifiers; large print or 'talking' clocks, watches and calculators; large numbered or automatic telephone dialers; specialized cooking equipment and other adaptive devices designed to enhance independence. Similarly, there are a variety of devices that are useful for the individual with a moderate to marked loss of hearing, despite the use of a hearing aid. Such devices include: digital alarm clocks with attachments that vibrate the pillow or bed when the alarm goes off;

telephone, television, radio, doorbell and smoke detector amplifiers; sound-activated strobe lights control; and closed-caption television decoders. For severe hearing loss or deafness, typewriter keyboards coupled with telephone receivers (TTDs), may be used to electronically transmit messages. 'Hearing dogs,' trained to respond to specific sounds and guide their mistresses to the source of those sounds, are also available to the deaf and profoundly hearing impaired.

While adaptive devices and equipment have the potential to maximize independence and quality of life, such aids are seldom covered by Medicare, Medicaid or private insurance. Given the prevalence of poverty among older women, many women have difficulty paying for adaptive aids that have the potential to make their adjustment process less stressful and isolating. Health care and human service providers need to look beyond traditional pay sources and resource agencies in order to help older women procure needed adaptive tools. It may be necessary to approach businesses, church groups, and civic organizations for their charitable assistance. Even simple replacement items such as hearing aid batteries can be cost prohibitive for some older women.

Transportation is a common problem for the older woman, particularly if she has a significant sensory impairment. Unmet transportation needs can have psychological implications as well: the lack of transportation may lead to increased dependency, isolation, hopelessness and a poor self-concept (Welsh, 1980). Private and public transportation resources available in the community should be explored, keeping in mind the woman's level of functional independence. While one woman may be able to independently use public transportation or a cab, another might need an attendant to assist with the visual or auditory demands outside her familiar environment. Supportive services, such as homemaker/chore services and home delivered meals are particularly useful to the visually impaired older woman who is unable to see well enough to effectively and safely cook or clean.

The use of any adaptive devices or concrete resources and services should be consciously designed and individually tailored to optimize functioning, reduce dependency and alleviate stress in order to enhance the older woman's sense of personal control and well-being.

When the nature of the impairment is progressive, the older woman's ongoing needs should be periodically reevaluated. This is particularly true in relation to eyeglass and hearing aid reevaluations.

Personal Control

Sensory impairment can be the precipitating factor for a variety of psychological and social problems. The concept of locus of control has significant implications related to adjustment and adaptation to sensory loss. Women who attribute their successes to internal causes affirm more pride and satisfaction in their accomplishments than do those who attribute success to an external cause. The literature reveals that internal locus of control is related to positive personal adjustment while external locus of control is associated with decreased psychosocial adjustment and health status. Vision and hearing limitations are both associated with situational unpredictability and personal vulnerability, reducing the woman's perception of personal control over her life. Unless she actively retains and cultivates her sense of personal control, the overwhelming psychosocial implications of vision or hearing impairment may result in loss of personal control for the older woman.

Research involving locus of control and hearing impaired individuals suggests that hearing impaired individuals tend to be more externally oriented than their hearing peers (Luckner, 1989). Similarly, the visually impaired are often regarded as dependent upon others, even when their assistive needs are relatively limited (Tuttle, 1984). Family members and friends may try to place the impaired older woman in a sort of 'protective capsule,' insulating her from many previous social roles, responsibilities and activities (Ainlay, 1988).

Even with the best adaptive behaviors and coping skills, those with significant vision or hearing loss are not totally self-sufficient: they must rely on the sighted or hearing to meet some needs. Decisions may be made for the woman without consulting her, thus limiting opportunities to utilize her decision-making and coping skills. Being frequently placed in a position of dependency on others may interfere with the sensory-impaired woman's natural drive toward self-sufficiency and autonomy. Unable to perceive alternate courses of action in a situation, she is limited to the one first discovered, or perhaps the course of action identified as best by significant others. While well-intentioned, the condescending actions of family and friends may have the tendency to exclude and alienate the older woman from the mainstream of daily life, casting her in the role of a secondary player in her own life and environment.

It is essential for both older women and involved professionals to understand that the concept of personal control is susceptible to positive as well as negative influence. Particularly potent in restoring a sense of personal control, cognitive and action oriented therapies allow the individual to encounter experiences that meaningfully alter her perception of the causality between personal actions and outcomes. To the maximum degree possible, the older woman should be allowed and encouraged to participate in the definition and planning of her health care, daily living and supportive service needs. Intervention goals and activities should relate to her day-to-day life, with an aim toward enhancing self-esteem and her acceptance of and adaptation to the sensory loss. Other aspects of personal adjustment or family functioning that interfere with the woman's independence should be addressed in order to empower her to overcome obstacles and develop constructive responses to the frustration associated with sensory loss. Family members may need to be encouraged to formulate and maintain realistic expectations that are commensurate with the older woman's wishes, needs and functional abilities.

Arranging for rehabilitation services is perhaps the most critical step toward maximizing function and the older woman's sense of personal control over her situation. Assisting her to realistically assess needs, capabilities and limitations enables her to objectively identify those tasks and decisions that require assistance and those that can be conducted independently. Without intervention, low self-confidence and diminished expectations for personal success may become self-fulfilling prophecies for the older woman with sensory impairments.

Social Support System

While the social needs of the sensory impaired women are the same as those of her sighted or hearing counterparts, the isolation and discomfort experienced in social settings may prompt her to withdraw physically and emotionally, as well as socially. At highest risk for social isolation are people who are single and live alone or who lack a supportive partner (Becker, 1981).

The social isolation of the visually and hearing impaired is well-substantiated (Schulz, 1972; Schulz, 1980; Tuttle, 1984; Demorest & Erdman, 1989). Yet, older women who are socially isolated are at considerable risk for avoidable or premature decline of both physical functioning and psychological well-being. Social support can mediate the negative effects and stressful situations associated with the sensory impairment. Studies reveal that individuals' reports of effective coping and low levels of psychological distress are associated with high levels of perceived support.

Professional intervention related to the sensory impaired woman's support system should include assessment of the adequacy of and her satisfaction with the existing social network. A particularly useful intervention involves facilitating the older woman's ability to assertively request needed assistance and constructively decline assistance that is unwarranted or undesired. Participation of family and close friends in counseling and rehabilitative efforts can strengthen communication patterns and support, while diminishing the older woman's feelings of isolation and resentment.

Upon identifying the strengths and limitations of the woman's informal support network, it may be pertinent to expand the network to include formal resources for purposes of both support and socialization. Formal resources include independent living services, church or community organizations that reflect the woman's interests and self-help or client advocacy groups. Mutual support groups are often particularly helpful in providing additional support or a replacement for social networks weakened after the onset of significant impairment.

Conscientious utilization of resources serves to provide sensory-impaired women with support, practical advice and important opportunities for socialization. In turn, these components can bring about improved self-concept, a greater sense of personal control and increased motivation. Furthermore, the utilization of formal resources often provides the family with needed physical and emotional support, reducing the stress associated with caregiving. If the nature of the older woman's sensory impairment is progressive, periodic reevaluation of her needs and satisfaction related to services provided by the informal and formal support networks is critical.

CONCLUSION

Because elderly women sometimes erroneously accept vision and hearing loss as inevitable and uncorrectable processes of aging, it is pertinent for the professional to encourage medical evaluation. If the sensory loss cannot be appreciably minimized, targeted efforts are indicated to facilitate the ability to constructively cope with and adapt to the limitations imposed by the loss. The professional's knowledge of appropriate restorative and rehabilitative services is essential in ensuring that the elderly woman's functional abilities are maximized. Adaptive devices, equipment and services designed to enhance independence, quality of life and safety are also essential ingredients for productive living and aging.

A sensory loss can be conceptualized as a stressful life event, correlated with increased levels of psychosocial distress and depression. Sensory loss late in life is commonly associated with a sense of personal loss, role changes, uncertainty regarding short- and long-term needs for adjustment, ambiguity concerning the new status and uncertainty regarding the reactions of significant others. Realistically, the impact of hearing loss includes not only the degree of its severity, but also the modifications in behavior that accompany the loss and the patient's capacity to adjust to the loss. When the sensory impairment is combined with concurrent functional limitations, the motivation for the older woman to learn important coping and maintenance skills may be diminished. Accordingly, adapting to and coping successfully with the problems and limitations associated with sensory loss may require significant effort and adjustment on her part. Individually tailored strategies designed to maximize the older woman's function, her sense of personal control, and her social support system can mediate the negative effects of sensory loss.

Over the past several decades, the outlook for the sensory impaired has dramatically improved, due to advances in medical knowledge, new surgical techniques, high performance vision and hearing aids and greater public awareness of available help. There is no question that intervention by multiple professions is an integral part of enabling older women to live productively with sensory loss.

REFERENCES

Ainlay, S. C. (1988). Aging and new vision loss: disruptions of the here and now. Journal of Social Issues, 44(1), pp. 79-94.

Alliance for Aging Research (1992). Independence for older Americans: Real answers to health & aging. Washington, DC: Author.

Barlow, E.; Siegal, D. L.; Edwards, F., & Doress, P. B. (1987). "Vision changes" in P. B. Doress, D. L. Siegal, & the Mildlife and Older Women Book Project (eds.), Ourselves, growing older, pp. 365-372. New York, NY: Simon and Schuster.

Barlow, E.; Doress, P. B., & Siegal, D. L. (1987). "Hearing impairment in the older years" in P. B. Doress, D. L. Siegal, & the Mildlife and Older Women Book Project (eds.), Ourselves, growing older, pp. 373-379. New York, NY: Simon and Schuster.

Beck, R. L. (1989). Hearing-impaired social workers: something lost, something gained. Social Work, Vol. 34(2), pp. 151-153.

Becker, G. (1981). Coping with stigma: Lifelong adjustment of deaf people. Social Science and Medicine, 15B, pp. 21-24.

Bess, F. H.; Lichenstein, M. J.; Logan, S. A., & Burger, C. M. (1989). Comparing criteria of hearing impairment in the elderly: a functional approach. Journal of Speech & Hearing Research, Vol. 32(4), pp. 795-802.

Better Hearing Institute. (1989). "You should hear what you're missing" (information packet/brochure). Washington, DC: Author.

Braille Institute (n.d.). Helping the blind to help themselves (pamphlet). Los Angeles, CA: Author.

Branch, L. G.; Horowitz, A., & Carr, C. (1989). The implications for everyday life of incident self-reported visual decline among people age 65 living in the community. The Gerontological Society of America, 29(3), pp. 359-365.

Commission on Education of the Deaf (1988). Toward equality: Education of the deaf. Washington, DC: U.S. Government Printing Office.

Demorest, M. E. & Erdman, S. A. (1989). Factor structure of the communication profile for the hearing impaired. Journal of Speech and Hearing Disorders, 54, pp. 541-549.

Ebersole, P. & Hess, P. (1981). Toward healthy aging. St. Louis: Mosby.

Greig, D. E.; West, M. L., & Overbury, O. (1986). Successful use of low vision aids: visual and psychological factors. Journal of Visual Impairment and Blindness, 80, pp. 985-988.

Kirchner, C. (1985). Data on blindness and visual impairment in the U.S.: a resource manual on characteristics, education, employment, and service delivery. New York, NY: American Foundation for the Blind.

Kirchner, C. & Lowman, C. (1978). Sources of variation in estimated prevalence of visual loss. Journal of Visual Impairment and Blindness, 72, pp. 267-270.

Luckman, J. & Sorenson, K. (1987). Medical surgical nursing: A psychophysiological approach. Philadelphia, PA: W. B. Saunders.

Luckner, J. L. (1989). Altering locus of control of individuals with hearing impairments by outdoor-adventure courses. Journal of Rehabilitation, 55(2), pp. 62-67.

National Center for Health Statistics (1982). Prevalence of selected physical impairments, by age, for persons 45 years and over: United States, 1979. Unpublished data. Cited in Special Committee on Aging, United States Senate, *Health and extended worklife.* Washington, DC: U.S. Government Printing Office.

National Hearing Aid Society (1988). The world of sound: Facts about hearing and hearing aids (booklet). Livonia, MI: Author.

National Institute on Aging (1987). The aging woman. Washington, DC: U.S. Department of Health and Human Services.

National Institute on Aging (1988). Special report on aging: 1987. Administrative document. Washington, DC: U.S. Government Printing Office.

Pearson, B. P. & Beck, C. M. (1989). Physical health of elderly women. Journal of Women & Aging, Vol. 1(1/2/3), pp. 149-174.

Schoenborn, C. A. & Morano, M. (1988). Current estimates from the national health interview survey: United States, 1977 (Vital Health Statistics, Series 10, No. 166, DHHS Publication No. PHS 88-1594). Washington, DC: U. S. Government Printing Office.

Schulz, P. (1972). Psychological factors in orientation and mobility training. New Outlook for the Blind, 66, pp. 129-134.

Schulz, P. (1980). How does it feel to be blind? Van Nuys, CA: Muse-Ed.

Tuttle, D. W. (1984). Self-esteem and adjusting with blindness: The process of responding to life's demands. Springfield, IL: Charles C Thomas, Publisher.

United States Senate Special Committee on Aging (1991). Developments in aging: 1990 (rept. 102-28, volumes 1 & 2). Washington, DC: United States Government Printing Office.

Welsh, R. L. (1980). Psychosocial dimensions. In R. L. Welsh & B. Blasch (eds.), Foundations of orientation and mobility. New York, NY: American Foundation for the Blind.

Wineburg, R. J. (1984). Geriatric blindness: a neglected public health problem. Health and Social Work, 9(1), pp. 36-41.

Discrimination Against Older Women in Health Care

Linda Liska Belgrave, PhD

SUMMARY. Growing awareness of apparent gaps in health care received by women and men raises concern over possible discrimination. This literature review examines this issue for elderly women, whose health care is obtained in a system that also may be permeated with age discrimination. Physicians tend to spend more time with women and older patients, suggesting that discrimination may not be an issue in the physician-patient relationship or may work in favor of older women. However, this may simply reflect elderly women's poorer health. Gender and age disparities in medical treatments received provide a more compelling argument that the health care system is a source of discrimination against older women, who are less likely than others to receive available treatments for cardiac, renal, and other conditions. The history of medical treatment of menopause suggests that stereotypes of older women have been advantageous for segments of the health care system. Finally, in addition to discrimination that has its source within the health care system itself, societal-wide inequities, particularly economic, are extremely detrimental to older women's health care. As we respond to the health care crisis, we must be alert to the potential to rectify those structures and tendencies that can lead to discrimination against women and the aged. Health care reform presents a unique opportunity to ensure health care equity.

Linda Liska Belgrave is affiliated with the Department of Sociology at the University of Miami, Coral Gables, FL.

[Haworth co-indexing entry note]: "Discrimination Against Older Women in Health Care." Belgrave, Linda Liska. Co-published simultaneously in the *Journal of Women & Aging* (The Haworth Press, Inc.) Vol. 5, No. 3/4, 1993, pp. 181-199; and: *Women and Healthy Aging: Living Productively in Spite of It All* (ed: J. Dianne Garner, and Alice A. Young), The Haworth Press, Inc., 1993, pp. 181-199. Multiple copies of this article/chapter may be purchased from The Haworth Document Delivery Center [1-800-3-HAWORTH; 9:00 a.m.-5:00 p.m. (EST)].

181

INTRODUCTION

Among the elderly, gender differences in the use of health care services are well documented, as are differences in the health problems experienced by older women and men. Currently, there is growing concern over the possibility that women and men receive different care for the same health problems. While differences do not necessarily indicate discrimination, this possibility must certainly be considered. This review addresses gender discrimination in the health care of the elderly at both the interpersonal and institutional levels. For this assessment, it is useful to distinguish between the health care system as a *source* of discrimination against older women and the receipt (or lack thereof) of health care as yet another instance of the negative impact of broader societal discrimination against women and the elderly. Because women's health in old age does not occur in a void, but reflects earlier health experiences, any assessment of this problem must take into account health care discrimination against younger women, as well as that against the elderly in general.

Health, Illness and Health Care Among the Elderly

Gender differences in health among the elderly extend well beyond women's well-known greater longevity. Although the leading causes of death are the same for older women and men, with some difference in ranking, at all ages beyond 65 men have higher mortality rates than women, a finding that holds for both whites and minorities. These mortality rates are reflected in life expectancy; at age 65 women can anticipate another 18 years, while men have only 14 years left, on average (Verbrugge, 1984). However, women's lower mortality and longer lives do not necessarily mean better health in old age.

Older women and men tend to give similar self-reports of their general health, but they experience significantly different health problems. While the elderly generally have fewer acute illnesses than do younger people, among the aged women have more acute illnesses and injuries than men. Older women also have more bed-disability days due to injury than older men, but it is unclear whether this is due to severity of injury, gender differences in response to injury or women's greater age (Verbrugge, 1984; Muller, 1990). In her analysis of multiple health surveys and other data sources, Verbrugge (1984) found that although older men are prone to more life-threatening ailments, elderly women tend to have more chronic health problems and to suffer more symptoms and physical limitations in their day-to-day lives. Arthritis, in particular, strikes and limits the activities of significantly more elderly women than men, while men are more likely to be limited by heart conditions. Verbrugge concluded, in part, that

> In one sense, older women have poorer health status than older men do because their daily lives are more troubled by symptoms (acute as well as chronic) and they find it more difficult to perform their social, physical, and mobility activities. . . . Ultimately, women die from the same diseases as men do, but at later ages. The delay allows them to accumulate nonkiller conditions, which often cause more daily bother than any "killer" conditions they have. (1984:314)

These gender differences in health reflect, in part, the health, work and family histories of today's elderly and may change as future cohorts reach old age (Verbrugge, 1984; Muller, 1990).

Older women and men differ not only in the nature of the health problems they experience, but also in their responses to these conditions. Using available literature and data to analyze gender differences in utilization of health care services, Muller (1990) determined that women's greater use of services continues into old age. Elderly women are more likely than male age peers to have visited a physician in the past year and have more physician visits during a year than men, a finding that also holds for widows and widowers. The use of preventive services follows this trend as well, with women having slightly more visits than men for physical exams, blood pressure checks and other such services. Men are more often hospitalized and undergo more procedures in the hospital, but women tend to have longer stays (Muller, 1990). Institutionalization, of course, plays a special role in the health care of elderly persons. Women's use of this form of care is considerably higher than men's. Older women are much more likely than older men to be institutionalized, have substantially longer lengths of stay and fill the vast majority of nursing home beds (Muller, 1990).

Older women's greater use of medical and other health care services when compared to men is, on the face of it, consistent with their greater incidence of and limitations from chronic health problems. Furthermore, the pattern whereby men are more frequently hospitalized, although for shorter stays, and receive more procedures is also unsurprising, given their greater incidence of life-threatening conditions. However, chronic condition incidence rates and health service utilization rates alone are not sufficient to determine whether there is equity in the delivery of health care. It is possible that gender differences in the health of the elderly should produce greater differences in health care. At the same time, it may well be that elderly women and men are both underserved, at least in part because of ageism (Muller, 1990).

THE HEALTH CARE SYSTEM
AS A SOURCE OF DISCRIMINATION

Growing interest in the possible effects of gender and age on health care is reflected in a rather diverse literature. In some instances, gender and/or age is simply included among many demographic variables in research with a different or broader focus (e.g., Hall, Roter & Katz, 1988). In other cases gender differences in physician-patient communications or in treatment constitute the research problem (e.g., Armitage, Schneiderman & Bass, 1979; Roter, Lipkin & Korsgard, 1991; Steingart et al., 1991). Age effects may or may not be addressed in such work. Finally, some authors address women's health care itself, without explicit comparison to that of men (e.g., Malterud, 1987), or focus on a condition that only women experience (e.g., McCrea, 1983). Together, these varied works begin to provide a picture of the ways in which older women are treated by the health care system.

Physician-Patient Interactions

The medical encounter itself provides a useful starting point in trying to understand gender and age differences in medical treatment. To the extent that physicians tend to stereotype patients by gender and age or to interact differently with women patients than with men, there is a potential for bias in medical conclusions drawn and treatments provided. The gender of the physician may also be relevant.

The literature on the relationship between patient gender and physician-patient communication contains findings that are seemingly contrary to "common sense" expectations of discrimination against women and in some cases, contradictory between studies. In his analysis of tape recorded (both audio and video) physician-patient interactions, Waitzkin (1985) found that physicians tended to spend more time with their female patients and gave them more explanations than their male patients. Older patients also received more explanations than others, although middle-aged patients tended to receive more of the physicians' time. These gender findings were confirmed in a meta-analysis of 41 published studies (Hall, Roter & Katz, 1988), which also found that providers gave somewhat more information to older patients. Furthermore, that analysis found that physicians provided more positive talk to women patients and were more likely to interrupt interviews with men by leaving the room. A more recent study, however, found that physicians made more statements to male than female patients (Roter, Lipkin & Korsgard, 1991). The inclusion of physician gender in the analysis showed that while men had longer visits than women when seeing male physicians, the reverse was true for female physicians. In addition, women physicians spent more time with their patients in general than did their male counterparts. In fact, physician gender had a stronger influence than patient gender on communication (Roter, Lipkin & Korsgard, 1991).

Studies of gender differences in physicians' responses to patients' medical complaints yield contradictory findings. Armitage, Schneiderman and Bass (1979) examined the medical records of 104 established patients with new complaints of back pain, headache, dizziness, chest pain and fatigue, a total of 181 visits. They found more extensive work-ups for male than female patients for all five of these common complaints. The differences were particularly striking for low back pain and headache. Using data from the National Ambulatory Medical Care Survey, Verbrugge and Steiner (1981) replicated and extended this work with a considerably larger sample (46,868 visits) and 15 groups of patient medical complaints. They found that women patients received more services per visit and more extensive services, particularly lab tests and blood pressure checks. In terms of the complaints examined by Armitage et al., women received more services for fatigue, chest pain and back pain, while men received more for vertigo and dizziness. When age and other variables were controlled in analysis, gender differences decreased for chest pain and fatigue, but increased for headache. Interestingly, women were more likely than men to be told to make an appointment for a follow-up visit, while men tended to be told to make a follow-up visit if necessary and were more likely to be referred to a specialist or hospital. The difference in the nature of the samples used for these two studies provides a likely partial explanation for the contradictory findings. However, it would be unwise to use the national study to dismiss Armitage, Schneiderman and Bass' (1979) results as simply a local phenomenon. Rather, the nature of the discrepancy suggests that there might be considerable variability in the ways in which physicians respond to similar complaints from male and female patients. Furthermore, while both of these studies found evidence of differential treatment for women and men (albeit conflicting differences), neither one conclusively answers the question of physician discrimination against women. The difficulty, of course, lies in trying to define such discrimination. For example, Verbrugge and Steiner's (1981) finding that women were likely to be told to make a follow-up appointment while men were more likely to be told to do so if they found it necessary could be interpreted as indicating that women were less likely to be treated as capable of determining their own need for a return visit. Women's higher average receipt of services might represent better care or simply greater susceptibility to provider created demand. More is not necessarily better.

Physician gender and the gender congruency between patient and provider may be relevant to treatment differences between women and men. In their review article, Weisman and Teitelbaum (1985) argue that physician gender would likely operate through effects on the physician-patient relationship, with particular emphasis on the attitudes and expectations of both physician and patient. Women physicians have been found to be more interested in interpersonal relationships while their male colleagues are more oriented toward science and research. Women physicians are more sensitive to issues of discrimination and to gender roles. However, male and female physicians are equally likely to conclude that women's problems are psychosomatic more often than men's. For their part, patients appear to view women physicians as more expressive than male physicians. In the same vein, Waller (1988) distinguishes three aspects of the physician-patient relationship that are potentially influenced by physician gender, including communication, affective tone and negotiative quality. The basic orientation of these authors, that physicians come to the relationship with past sex-role socialization and patients may well carry sex-role expectations of the physician, illuminates the processes through which gender influences physician-patient relationship, although the issue of relative power and authority in that relationship is not adequately addressed. This issue is particularly relevant when considering older women patients, who are likely to be at a greater disadvantage in the patient role than younger women, and considerably more so when compared to men of any age.

To what extent does physician gender influence treatments provided to women patients? A small Swiss study found women gynecologists to perform only half as many hysterectomies as their male colleagues (Domenightetti, Luraschi & Marazzi, 1985). Patient age was not addressed by the authors. The investigators suggested this difference may be due to the women physicians' greater understanding of their female patients' feelings about this emotionally charged surgery or to characteristics of women who seek female gynecologists.

Studies of the effect of physician-patient gender congruency on physical examinations yield less conclusive findings. Link and Zabar (1991) reviewed the charts of 529 patients to examine this issue in an urban teaching hospital clinic. They found that breast, genitourinary and rectal exams were not performed more frequently when physicians and patients were of the same gender. Unfortunately, the authors did not examine the effects of either patient or physician gender alone and potential effects of patient age were not analyzed. A similar, although smaller (N of 136 patients), study of cancer screening by family practice residents focussed on patients aged 50 and older (Levy, Dowling, Boult, Monroe & McQuade, 1992). In this case, male physicians were more likely than females to offer rectal exams to men aged 70 and older. Women doctors, on the other hand, were more likely than men to offer mammograms, pelvic exams and PAP smears to their women patients. This difference was particularly striking for patients age 50 to 70, to whom women physicians were 33% more likely to offer PAP smears than were their male colleagues. While the authors did not compare the receipt of cancer screening overall by patient gender, their report did contain some of the necessary data. Male and female patients were equally likely to have been offered rectal exams and fecal occult blood tests. While the literature regarding the effects of physician gender on older women's health care is not definitive, it does suggest that in some instances male and female physicians provide different levels of care to both genders. To the extent that women are underrepresented in medicine, women patients may be receiving inadequate care.

The relative absence of women in medicine, particularly in the development of this field and its basic concepts, may have even graver implications for women's health. The fact that the majority of patients with ill-defined problems are women suggests that the medical community has a poor understanding of women's health problems, resulting from "diagnostic narrowmindedness" (Malterud, 1987:207). The medical community's focus on organic disease rather than illness, and the classification schemes used for diagnosis may provide more confusion than enlightenment for women's health problems. This is, of course, confounded by the failure to include female subjects in major medical research (Katz, 1988) and the tendency to view the world from a male perspective (Wallis & Klass, 1990). Clearly, the dominance of the medical profession by men has contributed to this problem.

Medical Treatment

Much of the growing evidence that women and men receive different attention and care when experiencing similar health problems has come from epidemiological and other studies of specific ailments. Although the potential influence of patient age is not consistently examined in such work, coronary conditions, renal disease, hypertension and the use of tranquilizers and hypnotics are particularly relevant for an assessment of discrimination against older women. Despite the facts that diseases of the heart are the leading cause of death for both genders and that women have been found to have higher mortality rates than men 48 months after myocardial infarction (MI), women are less likely than men to be referred for cardiac catheterization and coronary bypass surgery (Steingart et al., 1991; Tofler et al., 1987; Tobin et al., 1987). While there has been evidence that results of stress tests might have to be interpreted differently for women than men (e.g., Sketch, Mohiuddin, Lynch, Zencka & Runco, 1975), such differences do not seem sufficient to justify the gender gap in testing and treatment. In a study of follow-up after exercise testing, Tobin et al. (1987) found that men were more than six times as likely as women to be referred for cardiac catheterization, even when controlling for medically relevant variables such as the test results, age, types of angina, symptoms and previous MI; the actual male/female rate of coronary artery disease was only 2:1. Myths that women have a greater tolerance for angina, that chest pain is benign in women and that stress tests are less effective for women than men have been cited as part of the explanation for gender disparities in treatments for heart problems (Steingart et al., 1991; Wenger, 1990). At least one author feels that coronary disease is simply believed to be less important in women and, therefore, is less vigorously treated (Katz, 1988). It is important to realize that these differences might reflect either under use of catheterization and by-pass surgery for women or overuse of such techniques for men (Steingart et al., 1991). Either way, these and other findings indicate clear inequities in care that must be examined and rectified.

Gender and age disparities have also been found in the use of chronic renal dialysis and renal transplantation. Using national data for 1979 Kjellstrand and Logan (1987) found that 37% of men in need of renal dialysis received this treatment, but only 31% of women, a statistically significant difference. While half of those aged 55-64 needing dialysis received it, this was true for only 33% of those aged 65-74 and a mere 6% for those 75 or older. Among whites, the fraction treated was higher for women than men at ages

45-64, but lower for all other ages. Among African Americans the pattern differed; women had higher treatment rates than men during childhood and early adulthood (through age 24) and at 65 or older. African Americans had lower treatment rates at all ages below 65. An analysis of renal transplant based on national data for 1983 and midwest data for 1979-1985 showed that the transplant rate for women aged 45-60 was less than half the rate for male age and race peers (Kjellstrand, 1988). Even when adjusting for cytotoxic antibodies (higher for women), men had an advantage in terms of transplant. The midwest data showed the inequality to be consistent over time.

The use of tranquilizers in long-term care facilities and of hypnotic drugs for sleeplessness among the elderly are of particular concern. A secondary analysis of data from a 300 bed facility found that women were more likely than men to be treated with tranquilizers. Women were more likely than men to be defined as anxious and among anxious patients, women were more than five times as likely as men to be on tranquilizers (Milliren, 1977). Men, on the other hand, were more likely to be treated with tranquilizers if they scored low in mental status or were unfriendly to staff, while these two variables did not influence treatment for women. A British study of the use of hypnotic drugs (mostly benzodiazepine) for sleep by the elderly living in the community found that women were more likely to use such medications (Morgan, Dallosso, Ebrahim, Arie & Fentem, 1988). Furthermore, the level of use increased with age for women, but not for men. Nearly three-quarters of the sample had been using hyponotics for over a year and one quarter for over ten years. Given that these drugs lose their sleep-inducing effects within two weeks of continuous use, overuse was clearly a problem. To the extent that this was more common among women than men, women were more likely to be receiving poor medical advice. Although patterns of use of hypnotic medications found among a British sample cannot be generalized directly to the U.S., these findings do suggest the need to examine this issue here.

Not all gender differences in testing for and treating health problems result in less favorable outcomes for women. A study of medical records in a rural community health clinic found that the rates of detection of hypertension were better for women than for men, as well as for the elderly compared to the young (Doyle, Lauterbach, Samargo, Robinson & Ludwig, 1991).

An examination of conditions experienced only by women can demonstrate the ways in which sexism and ageism permeate the health care system. Among women, older age can influence the care received for health problems that can occur at any age. For instance, older women appear less likely than their younger peers to receive appropriate care for breast cancer (Muller, 1990). The possible contributions to this situation of stereotypes and economic factors cannot be ignored. Given medicine's historical tendency to define women's health in reproductive terms and the resultant view of older women as useless and somehow not really women (Vertinsky, 1988), it would not be surprising to see ageism in women's health care manifested in health problems related to reproduction and/or sexuality. Compounding this potential problem is the issue of economics. Older women's reliance on Medicare or a combination of Medicare and Medicaid, when compared to younger women's more likely coverage by private health insurance, may well reduce the financial rewards of appropriate treatment or even throw up barriers in the way of health care providers.

Medical handling of menopause suggests that gender and age stereotypes are potentially beneficial for segments of the health care industry. Although menopause is typically acknowledged to be a normal, natural part of the aging process, it is at the same time treated as an abnormality, a disease. Women are referred to labs for hormone tests so "diagnoses" can be made and "treatment" options discussed. In her analysis, McCrea (1983) traced early definitions of menopause through the current approach. During the Victorian era, menopause was seen as a sign of "sin and decay." With the Freudian influence of the early twentieth century, this conception changed and menopause came to be seen as a neurosis. The advent of synthetic hormones in the 1960s brought a dramatic change in the medical view of menopause. The pharmaceutical industry had developed a readily available treatment in need of a disease. The medical community found that disease in menopause, which became defined as a deficiency disease, the treatment for which was estrogen replacement therapy (ERT). In 1975 half of all post-menopausal women had used ERT at least temporarily; the median length of use was 10 years. Although the use of estrogen dropped with the discovery at that time of a link between ERT and endometrial cancer, it was still overprescribed. McCrea's (1983) analysis clearly demonstrates the use of cultural stereotypes of older women as useless and repulsive in the medicalization of menopause. Her analysis also suggests, but does not examine in detail, the manipulation of these stereotypes by the pharmaceutical industry for the sake of profits and by physicians to fill waiting rooms. The use of ERT remains controversial. The benefits claimed for this therapy (e.g., relief from hot flashes and vaginal dryness and prevention of osteoporosis) have become more modest in light of the risks (Boston Women's Health Book Collective, 1984), but some still advise that

> . . . *all women* should be treated as probable victims [of osteoporosis], regardless of radiographic evaluation . . . estrogens should begin soon after the diagnosis of menopause [in women who do not have contraindications], regardless of symptoms. (DeFazio & Speroff, 1985:42)

Given the cloud of uncertainty introduced by the role of vested interests in this controversy and recommendations such as this, it is quite difficult to evaluate the possible benefits of ERT.

HEALTH CARE AS IT REFLECTS SOCIETAL DISCRIMINATION

The health care system, as part of the larger social structure, can present problems for older women not only as a source of age and gender discrimination, but also as an arena in which the effects of wider societal discrimination against women and the elderly are played out. The economic situations in which many elderly women find themselves and social policy regarding aging and health care are of particular importance.

It comes as no surprise that those age 65 and older have lower incomes than younger persons. In 1988 elderly men had a median annual income of $12,471, less than half that of men age 45 to 54 ($29,578). Although the percentage gap for women was not as great, incomes for both age groups were considerably lower, at

$12,020 for women age 45 to 54 and a mere $7,103 for old women (U.S. Bureau of the Census, 1991). Thus, on average, elderly women's income was only 57% of the income of elderly men, indicating a clear and dramatic disadvantage. In the mid 1980s the poverty rate for elderly women was 19% (Minkler & Stone, 1985) and nearly a quarter of poor women were age 60 or older (Wilson, 1987). Among unmarried white women the poverty rate was 31%, compared to 21% for male peers. Fully 69% of unmarried African American women and 49% of unmarried African American men were living in poverty (Minkler & Stone, 1985). Furthermore, elderly women are less likely than men to escape poverty (Coe, 1988). These gender differences are, of course, rooted in the long-term pattern of women's dependence on men, the sexual division of labor and economic discrimination against women in the work place. However, the feminization of poverty among the elderly was considerably exacerbated by the Federal Budget cuts of the early 1980s (Minkler & Stone, 1985). (Although the emphasis here is on gender discrimination, it is necessary to note that the racial differences above are considerably greater than those due to gender.)

Despite virtually universal Medicare coverage for those age 65 and older, access to health care and the quality of health care that is received are affected by the ability to pay co-payments and other out-of-pocket costs. The poorest of the elderly may be eligible for Medicaid, but eligibility requirements vary by state. Even where those requirements are fairly liberal, some will be in the position of not qualifying for Medicaid, yet unable to afford the cost-sharing required to use their Medicare benefits. Elderly in this position who rate their health as fair or poor use fewer physician services than others (Muller, 1990). Given their lower incomes, women are less likely to be able to afford private Medigap insurance. Among those elderly making physician visits, men do, in fact, appear to be somewhat more likely than women to pay for them using private insurance. Although there is little gender difference in the overall use of public sources, women are more likely to rely on Medicaid, with men using more veterans' benefits (Muller, 1990). Elderly women may be particularly vulnerable to the need to spend down into poverty in order to get Medicaid coverage for health care (Grau, 1987). What is unknown is the extent to which poor and near-poor elderly do without needed health care because they simply cannot afford it. Based on the income and poverty data above, it is clear that a greater proportion of elderly women than men are likely to be caught in this position.

The relationships between gender, poverty and lack of health care are exacerbated by the relationship between poverty and poor health. The poor of any age are more likely than others to suffer from poor health, a relationship that has been consistent over time (Syme & Berkman, 1990). This general relationship holds for the elderly as a whole and for elderly women. That is, among older women the poor tend to evaluate their health as poorer than do others and are more likely to report health-related limitations in their activities (Muller, 1990).

A more subtle problem is that of the time spent in obtaining care, a burden that falls disproportionately on both the poor and on women. The former may be seen as socially unimportant by health care providers and thus, kept waiting. Because the poor are kept waiting for so many services, these time constraints can pose very real problems. Women's time might be seen as more flexible than that of men, based on stereotypes of the housewife role, justifying burdensome waits for care (Gauthier, 1991). This problem may be shared by the elderly, based on care providers' perceptions of the leisure time available to retirees. As with the problems of poverty and financial access to care, this sort of time impediment, based in stereotypes, originates outside of the health care system and similar problems are undoubtedly seen in other social institutions. Nonetheless, when it is played out in a health care setting, the results are age and gender inequities in health care.

CONCLUSION

Older women and men experience qualitatively different patterns of health problems, with women suffering more day-to-day symptoms and limitations while men tend to develop life-threatening ailments. Likewise, the use of health care services by the elderly varies by gender. Older women have more physician visits whereas men experience more, and shorter, hospitalizations. Moreover, there is evidence that older women and men do not receive the same responses from their health care providers. Although differences in services provided do not, in and of themselves, indicate discrimination against older women, they do point to the need to examine this possibility.

Gender differences exist in communication and attention during office visits and possibly in patient work-ups and services provided. The greater amount of time spent by physicians with older and female patients suggests that gender discrimination may not be an issue in physician-elderly patient interaction, or may work in women's favor. However, such findings must be interpreted in the context of older women's health problems. As is the case in terms of health care utilization itself, this may simply reflect elderly women's greater incidence of chronic illness and greater limitations. Furthermore, to the extent that medicine is biased toward a male perspective, diagnostic categories may be inadequate for women's health problems and the "extra" office visit time spent with women may be used asking the wrong questions.

Gender and age disparities in medical treatments received provide an even more compelling argument for the existence of discrimination in health care. The gender gap in cardiac catheterization and by-pass surgery cannot be explained. Women in general and the elderly are less likely than others to receive renal dialysis, with an even greater disadvantage in terms of renal transplant. Older women are more likely than men to be treated with tranquilizers or hypnotic sleeping aids. Older women appear to receive less adequate care for breast cancer than their younger peers, a situation that may be related to stereotypes of elderly women. There is no question that medical handling of menopause has been, and continues to be, influenced by such stereotypes.

Discrimination against older women, or any other group, in health care does not occur in a social vacuum. Societal-wide inequities, particularly economic, have a tremendous impact on the health care received by older women. Elderly women are more likely than either younger women or aged men to be poor, and, because of their poverty, likely to be in worse health than others. At the same time, while older women's poverty doubtless increases their need for health care, relative to others, it decreases their ability to obtain such care. Although the sources of these problems are outside the health care system itself, the consequences are gender inequities in obtaining health care, a form of health care discrimination against older women.

Healthy Aging in the Face of Discrimination

Efforts to help older women avoid discrimination and to live well despite its existence can be directed to each of the levels at which inequities occur, including provider-patient interactions, medical treatment, research, and access to health care. At the most fundamental level, health care practitioners can learn to recognize the interference of gender and age stereotypes and expectations in interactions with, and treatment of, their own patients. Furthermore, they can help their patients recognize such influences, so that they will be better able to protect themselves in interactions with other professionals. In the same vein, practitioners can increase their attention to the shortcomings of current "knowledge" regarding women's aging. Obviously, treatment sometimes will have to be provided despite a lack of solid research with older women. Increased awareness of the extent to which this happens may help providers avoid unintended inappropriate differential treatment of older women and be more sensitive to these women's deviations from expectations based on male patients and research subjects. Sharing such evaluations of clinical research with patients would increase older women's ability to make informed decisions regarding treatment options.

The exclusion of women subjects from medical research and the resultant ignorance of appropriate treatments for women can and must be rectified by that segment of the health care system that determines research priorities (e.g., Federal funding agencies, pharmaceutical corporations, academics). Clearly, those conducting research must increase the inclusion of women in study samples and demand the same from colleagues less sensitive to this issue. Furthermore, using professional associations, publications and the like, practitioners can make known their needs for relevant research.

Solutions to broader forms of discrimination against older women in health care are beyond the health care system itself. The deplorable level of poverty among elderly women, particularly minority women, must be addressed at the societal level. A national health care plan that guaranteed service to all would go a long way toward eliminating discrimination in access to care. Certainly health care professionals should be actively engaged in efforts to expand the provision of health care to the disadvantaged. Furthermore, direct service providers, through their regular contact with patients and their problems, are in a unique position to draw older women into efforts to improve the health care system. Such involvement would not only increase the likelihood that health care reform would address the needs of older women, but would also empower them, increasing their ability to deal with discrimination when they experience it.

Given women's changing roles and increased presence in the labor force, future cohorts of elderly women are likely to approach the health care system from a stronger position than those now dealing with the problems outlined above. Current concern over the health care crisis suggests that tomorrow's elderly women are also likely to face a different health care system. As we struggle to change the ways in which health care is provided, we must be alert to the potential to rectify those structures and tendencies that can lead to discrimination against women and the aged. Health care reform presents a unique opportunity to ensure health care equity.

REFERENCES

Armitage, Karen J., Lawrence J. Schneiderman and Robert A. Bass. 1979. "Response of Physicians to Medical complaints in Men and Women." *Journal of the American Medical Association* 241:2186-2187.

Boston Women's Health Book Collective. 1984. *The New Our Bodies, Ourselves.* New York: Simon & Schuster.

Coe, Richard D. 1988. "A Longitudinal Examination of Poverty in the Elderly Years." *Gerontologist* 28:540-544.

DeFazio, John and Leon Speroff. 1985. "Estrogen Replacement Therapy: Current Thinking and Practice." *Geriatrics* 40: 32-37, 40-43, 47-48.

Domenightetti, Gianfranco, Pierangelo Luraschi and Alfio Marazzi. 1985. "Hysterectomy and Sex of the Gynecologist." *New England Journal of Medicine* 313:1482.

Doyle, Daniel B., Walt Lauterbach, Pat Samargo, Craig Robinson and William Ludwig. 1991. "Age- and Sex-Biased Underdetection of Hypertension in a Rural Clinic." *Family Practice Research Journal* 11:395-404.

Gauthier, Candace. 1991. "Time Demands and Medical Ethics in Women's Health Care." *Health Care for Women International* 12:153-165.

Grau, Lois. 1987. "Illness-Engendered Poverty Among the Elderly." *Women and Health* 12:103-118.

Hall, Judith A., Debra L. Roter and Nancy R. Katz. 1988. "Meta-analysis of Correlates of Provider Behavior in Medical Encounters." *Medical Care* 26:657-675.

Katz, Sidney. 1988. "More Effort to Solve 'Male Diseases' than Female Ones, MD Says." *Canadian Medical Association Journal* 139:65-66.

Kjellstrand, Carl M. and George M. Logan. 1987. "Racial, Sexual and Age Inequalities in Chronic Dialysis." *Nephron* 45:257-263.

Kjellstrand, Carl M. 1988. "Age, Sex and Race Inequality in Renal Transplantation." *Archives of Internal Medicine* 148:1305-1309.

Levy, Sheldon, Patrick Dowling, Lisa Boult, Alicia Monroe and William McQuade. 1992. "The Effect of Physician and Patient Gender on Preventive Medicine Practices in Patients Older Than Fifty." *Family Medicine* 24:58-61.

Link, R. Nathan and Sondra R. Zabar. 1991. "Physician-Patient Gender Congruence and the Physical Examination." *Journal of General Internal Medicine* 6:466-468.

Malterud, Kristi. 1987. "Illness and Disease in Female Patients." *Scandinavian Journal of Primary Health Care* 5:205-209.

McCrea, Frances B. 1983. "The Politics of Menopause: The 'Discovery' of a Deficiency Disease." *Social Problems* 31:111-123.

Milliren, John W. 1977. "Some Contingencies Affecting the Utilization of Tranquilizers in Long-Term Care of the Elderly." *Journal of Health and Social Behavior* 18:206-211.

Minkler, Meredith and Robyn Stone. 1985. "The Feminization of Poverty and Older Women." *Gerontologist* 25:351-357.

Morgan, Kevin, Helen Dallosso, Shah Ebrahim, Tom Arie and Peter H. Fentem. 1988. "Prevalence, Frequency, and Duration of Hypnotic Drug Use Among the Elderly Living at Home." *British Medical Journal* 296:601-602.

Muller, Charlotte F. 1990. *Health Care and Gender.* New York: Russell Sage.

Roter, Debra, Mack Lipkin and Audry Korsgard. 1991. "Sex Differences in Patients and Physicians Communication During Primary Care Medical Visits." *Medical Care* 29: 1083-1093.

Sketch, Michael H., Syed M. Mohiuddin, Joseph D. Lynch, Allen E. Zencka and Vincent Runco. 1975. "Significant Sex Difference in the Correlation of Electrocardiographic Exercise Testing and Coronary Arteriograms." *The American Journal of Cardiology* 36:169-173.

Steingart, Richard M., Milton Packer, Peggy Hamm, Mary Ellen Coglianese, Bernard Gersh, Edward M. Geltman, Josephine Sollano, Stanley Katz, Lem Moyé, Lofty L. Basta, Sandra J. Lewis, Stephen S. Gottlieb, Victoria Bernstein, Patricia McEwan, Kirk Jacobson, Edward J. Brown, Marrick L. Kukin, Niki E. Kantrowitz and Marc A. Pfeffer. 1991. "Sex Differences in the Management of Coronary Artery Disease." *New England Journal of Medicine* 325:226-230.

Syme, S. Leonard and Lisa F. Berkman. 1990. "Social Class, Susceptibility, and Sickness." Pgs. 28034 in Peter Conrad and Rochelle Kern (eds.) *The Sociology of Health & Illness: Critical Perspectives.* New York: St. Martins.

Tobin, Jonathan N., Sylvia Wassertheil-Smoller, John P. Wexler, Richard M. Steingart, Nancy Budner, Lloyd Lense and Joseph Wachspress. 1987. "Sex Bias in Considering Coronary Bypass Surgery." *Annals of Internal Medicine* 107:19-25.

Tofler, Geoffrey H., Peter H. Stone, James E. Muller, Stefan N. Willich, Vicki G. Davis, W. Kenneth Poole, H. William Strauss, James T. Willerson, Allan S. Jaffe, Thomas Robertson, Eugene Passamani, Eugene Braunwald and the Milis Study Group. 1987. "Effects of Gender and Race on Prognosis after Myocardial Infarction: Adverse Prognosis for Women, Particularly Black Women. *Journal of the American College of Cardiology* 9:473-482.

U.S. Bureau of the Census. 1991. *Statistical Abstract of the United States: 1991* (111th edition.) Washington, D.C.: U.S. Government Printing Office.

Verbrugge, Lois M. and Richard P. Steiner. 1981. "Physician Treatment of Men and Women Patients: Sex Bias or Appropriate Care?" *Medical Care* 19:609-632.

Verbrugge, Lois M. 1984. "A Health Profile of Older Women with Comparisons to Older Men." *Research on Aging* 6:291-322.

Vertinsky, Patricia. 1988. " 'Of No Use Without Health': Late Nineteenth Century Medical Prescriptions for Female Exercise through the Life Span." *Women and Health* 14:89-115.

Waitzkin, Howard. 1985. "Information Giving in Medical Care." *Journal of Health and Social Behavior* 26:81-101.

Waller, Kathy. 1988. "Women Doctors for Women Patients?" *British Journal of Medical Psychology* 61:125-135.

Wallis, Lila A. and Perri Klass. 1990. "Towards Improving Women's Health Care." *Journal of the American Medical Women's Association* 45:219-221.

Weisman, Carol S. and Martha Ann Teitelbaum. 1985. "Physician Gender and the Physician Patient Relationship: Recent Evidence and Relevant Questions." *Social Science and Medicine* 20:1119-1127.

Wenger, Nanette K. 1990. "Gender, Coronary Artery Disease, and Coronary Bypass Surgery." *Annals of Internal Medicine* 112:557-558.

Wilson, Julie Boatright. 1987. "Women and Poverty: A Demographic Overview." *Women and Health* 12:21-40.

Public Policy, Health Care
and Older Women

Lou Ann B. Jorgensen, DSW

SUMMARY. For the first time in history, long life has become a problem. The most serious problem facing the older generation is the availability and affordability of health care. While the life expectancy of both men and women continues to increase, the older population of the U.S. is becoming increasingly feminine. In the last two decades there has been a dramatic fall in poverty among the aged, yet for many elderly persons and especially older women, Social Security benefits barely keep them above the poverty level. Access to medical care has improved with Medicaid and Medicare, but not to the extent the aging population had anticipated. Proposals for universal health care have been put forth by politicians, legislators and professional organizations, some of which acknowledge the unique health problems of aging women while others are discriminatory to the aged in general and women in particular. Many believe women must assert themselves if their health care needs are to be adequately and fairly addressed. To this end, more women than ever are becoming involved in the political process, running for and being elected to local, state and national offices. It is anticipated that these women will be sensitive to the health care needs of older women and put forth efforts to develop and implement policies which address these needs.

INTRODUCTION

"The four generation family will become common," wrote Cynthia M. Taeuber, author of the 1991 Census Bureau report on Amer-

Lou Ann B. Jorgensen is Associate Dean, Graduate School of Social Work, University of Utah, Salt Lake City, UT 84112.

[Haworth co-indexing entry note]: "Public Policy, Health Care and Older Women." Jorgensen, Lou Ann B. Co-published simultaneously in the *Journal of Women & Aging* (The Haworth Press, Inc.) Vol. 5, No. 3/4, 1993, pp. 201-220; and: *Women and Healthy Aging: Living Productively in Spite of It All* (ed: J. Dianne Garner, and Alice A. Young), The Haworth Press, Inc., 1993, pp. 201-220. Multiple copies of this article/chapter may be purchased from The Haworth Document Delivery Center [1-800-3-HAWORTH; 9:00 a.m.-5:00 p.m. (EST)].

ica's elderly. "Children will know their grandparents and even their great-grandparents, especially their great-grandmothers. And more people will face the concern and expense of caring for their old, frail relatives, since so many people now live long enough to face multiple, chronic illnesses" (Taeuber, 1991).

This chapter will examine health care for older women and the public policies that affect and influence how the older woman can depend on receiving health care. For those who today are considered members of the older generation of either gender, female or male, or for those who will soon be among those in the older generation, the most serious problem this population will face is the availability of health care. This generation has grown up presuming health care is a basic human right and one they could rely on when needed during their entire lifetime. Today, we find this is not always true and especially for some specific populations, such as older women and the poor.

Some who influence public policy question that presumed right, often writing off the elderly because they do not believe health care is a right, or for that matter, necessary. The lack of consensus on whether health care is a right and that the community has an obligation to fulfill that right, may be one of the explanations of why we don't have a national health-care system or other means to assure the availability of health care for all. What can be done to assure that health care is available to all elderly persons, especially to aging women, who appear to have a longer life expectancy than men and will require health care for a longer period of time?

Health care for the aged American has been on the social policy agenda since the early twentieth century. The goals of social policy related to health care have always been to provide adequate health care while containing health care costs. Policy continues to focus on the provision of services and resources and how to implement those services and resources for the populations who need them while being fiscally responsible. As America grows and as the aged populations live longer, this agenda becomes more difficult to follow.

The population of the United States is aging and, among the old, becoming increasingly feminine. Life expectancy of females born in 1985 was 78.2, or seven years longer than that of men. The disparity between survival of men and women in the United States has widened significantly since the turn of the century (Rice, 1989). Projections from the "Middle Series" of the U.S. Bureau of the Census (1989) expect an increase in life expectancy of both men and women, with a continuation of the gender differential. Life expectancy at birth for men is projected to increase to 75 years by 2040 and for women to 83.1 years, a differential of 8.1 years. At age 65, life expectancy is projected to increase to 17.1 years for men and 22.6 years for women. Thus, if true, women's life expectancy in the future will be 87.6 or possibly higher.

The many layered family described in the 1991 Census Bureau report stems from the rapid growth of the number of Americans 65 or older. Largely as a result of medical and public health advances, that group grew by 22% during the 1980's, more than double the growth of the nation as a whole. And it will continue to grow: 50 years from now, the nation could have more people older than age 65 than young people aged 20 and younger, the study said. At the same time, the report counters the perception that most elderly are in poor health. Three-quarters of those aged 65 to 74 who are not living in institutions, say they are in good health. And even among those 75 and older, two-thirds consider themselves healthy (Taeuber, 1991).

Perhaps for the first time in history long life has become a problem. The old-old, being defined as persons eighty-five years of age and older, represented 1 percent of the U. S. population in 1980. According to Bureau of Census (1984) projections, they will be 1.8 of the population in 2000, 2.8 percent in 2030, and 5.9 percent in 2080. This group has chronic health problems and extraordinary social needs. Nearly one-fourth of the old-old are institutionalized, and one-half of those who are not institutionalized need someone else's help in order to cope with everyday life (Suzman & Reley, 1985). In its single-minded focus on extending life through technology, medicine has ignored the quality of life (Martin, 1990).

We know that in the past decade many Americans have sought to learn more about how they could improve their current and future health. Undoubtedly, many persons will avoid serious health problems with improved nutrition and fitness, but from much of the current research, we are aware that a percentage of the population will face serious health problems as they age. Women will be the highest percentage of that population and often women alone as they age. One-third of women in the United States are widowed by the time they reach age sixty-five. At age seventy-five well over half are widowed, and by eighty-five over 80 percent are (Holden, 1989).

Another factor of this aloneness for older women is the fact that because of our mobile society many women live in communities . . . "where members of their immediate family no longer reside." The immediate families of these women have often died before their sibling or they live in communities outside of the states where other family members reside. The children of these women, if they have children many (of whom) are aging themselves, have lived for many years away from the homes of their parents. And another generation, grandchildren, live at even greater distances. The main support systems of some older women become neighbors, members of their social or religious groups, or younger individuals who reside near them. One of the saddest scenarios of aging is when an older woman shares with you that all of her friends have now died so she has no one to relate to and she is becoming too old to travel to see her family. This can often be because of lack of funds rather than health reasons.

A major accomplishment of federal policy over the last two decades has been a dramatic fall in poverty among the aged. Social Security benefits have increased sufficiently to keep the incomes of many elderly and disabled persons from falling below the poverty line (Martin, 1990). In 1960 over one third of all individuals sixty-five years of age or older were counted as poor; by the mid-1980s that percentage had fallen to 12.4, a rate which has remained fairly constant since then. Although in 1960 poverty was far more prevalent among the elderly than for the general population (35.2 versus 22.4 percent, respectively, were poor), the percentage of the elderly who are poor is now less than that of the population (12.4 versus 13.6 percent, respectively) (Holden, 1988).

The Census Bureau (1991) report shows that of the 31.2 million persons over 65, 27.9% are white, 2.5% are black and 0.8 are defined as other. The poverty rates, while low overall, vary considerably by race and origin: of the group 10% were white, 34% were black and 23% Hispanic and other (Taeuber, 1991).

PUBLIC POLICY AND LEGISLATIVE TRENDS

U.S. health care is languishing in a debilitating condition, the main symptoms of which are runaway costs and a shameful lack of attention to many ill citizens. American society does not receive fair value for the vast sums of money it devotes to health care. The time is ripe for public policy initiatives to remedy this malady by creating the basis for a health-care system that is both more efficient and more effective (Martin, 1990).

National health policy in America presents many examples of the problems of rational policy making. Political issues intervene at every stage of the rational decision-making process–in defining the goals of health policy, in identifying alternative courses of action, in assessing their potential costs, and in selecting policy alternatives that maximize the quality and accessibility of health care while minimizing costs (DiNitto, 1991).

Health care is a basic human need. Most of us would argue that nobody should suffer because they lack the financial resources to obtain adequate medical attention. Prior to 1965, medical care for the poor was primarily a responsibility of state and local governments and private charity. But interest in national health care for the poor particularly dates back to the turn of the century, when reform groups during the Progressive Era first proposed a national health insurance plan. This continued to be discussed until 1935 when opposition from the American Medical Association (AMA) forced President Franklin D. Roosevelt to abandon the idea of including health insurance in the original Social Security Act for fear that it would endanger passage of the entire act (DiNitto, 1991).

Major health bills continued to be introduced into Congress every year from 1935 to 1965. In 1965 changes were made in the Social Security Act to provide health care to the poor and aged. Social Security is a prominent example of the success of comprehensive income security policy. What we need is a similarly successful minimum income policy. Many welfare states have a legislated universal minimum income policy, including West Germany (since 1961), the Netherlands (1963), the U.K. (1970), Belgium (1974), Israel (1980), Luxembourg (1986), and France (1986). The policies are intended to provide aid to families that are not covered by Social Security (Martin, 1990). If both of these plans were available older women may be covered with an opportunity to receive health care by one means or the other.

The growing cost of health care since 1960 is reflected in several measures. Between 1960 and 1985, the health expenditure share of GNP (Gross National Product) rose from 5.3 percent to 10.7 percent and per capita health expenditures from $146 to $1,721. Average annual expenditure increases have ranged from 8.9 to 15.7 percent, with the medical care price index of recent years rising almost three times as fast as the CPI (Consumer Price Index). Despite a huge real increase in the supply of key health care personnel and facilities, the average hospital cost per patient day has grown by about 400 percent since 1970, as has the average cost per patient stay (U.S. Bureau of the Census, 1986).

Entitlement programs under Social Security which were part of the Older American Act introduced Medicaid to address the health needs of the aging and those in need. Everyone who qualifies and needs assistance should be served. Medicare, as well as other amendments to the Social Security Act, provides prepaid hospital insurance for the aged under Social Security and low-cost medical insurance for the aged. Eligibility for Medicare does not depend on income while Medicaid recipients have a limitation on the amount of resources available to them. Access to medical care has improved with Medicaid and Medicare but not to the extent the aging population had anticipated. Many older persons acquire additional supplementary insurance to assure their health needs will be taken care of in later life. Many advertised supplementary health insurance plans should be studied thoroughly as they often do not provide the means to cover the additional costs of health needs.

From 1970 to 1985, direct public expenditures for health climbed from $28 billion to $175 billion. During that period, the federal share of these expenditures increased from 64 percent to 71 percent. Most of the nonfederal public expenditures involve state contributions to Medicaid and funding of state and local hospitals. On the federal side, about 60 percent of spending is devoted to Medicare payments, another 18 percent to the federal portion of Medicaid funding, 10 percent to public health activities, and 7 percent for the care of veterans. The remaining 5 percent is divided among medical research, hospital and medical costs for the Defense Department, child health programs, and other activities (U.S. Bureau of Census, 1987).

CONSUMER PLANS FOR HEALTH CARE

The landscape of American health care is marked by several contradictions. While the vast majority (85 percent) of Americans have easy access to a wide variety of medical services through employment-based insurance programs, Medicaid, or Medicare, some 35 million people are totally without coverage. Health care reform is the agenda item of the 90s. The national elections of November, 1992 saw politicians position health care as one of the top issues. The President and Vice President who were elected promised during campaigning that one of their first hundred-day agenda items was to address access to health care for all. If accomplished, aging women may find support and answers to how they will access their health care in the future.

Prior to the election, two organizations presented plans to assist in accessing health care for all Americans. The American Medical Association (AMA) in July of 1992 presented a plan prefaced by this statement pertaining to health access: "The status quo is unacceptable. We need control of health care costs. We need affordable health insurance for all Americans. Health care reform should build on the strengths of our uniquely American system of health care" (American Medical Association, 1992).

"Health Access America" is the AMA's action plan to restrain the growth of health care costs and provide affordable health insurance for all. The plan "preserves our ability to choose the care that is the best for us." Health Access America has four goals: cost containment, universal health insurance coverage, quality assurance, and freedom of choice. These goals are defined by the AMA in their Health Access America brochure made available to the public through public advertisements. They are suggesting that their goals are to be met to assist all Americans by containing health care costs. The plan is to reduce the spending of health dollars for insurance marketing and risk avoidance techniques; curb administrative costs and paperwork by using uniform claim forms and electronic billing; use "practice parameters" to assure health dollars are going to health care that is appropriate for each patient; reform professional liability laws to eliminate unnecessary "defensive" health services that protect against lawsuits but don't benefit patients.

AMA further states, "We can hold down health care costs by improving the market in which we buy health insurance and health services." This can be accomplished by fostering competition in the health care marketplace and empowering patients to make their own choices based on cost efficient care and reasonable insurance costs; and, encouraging wiser spending of health care dollars. AMA would encourage clients to ask the cost of medical procedures before they have the procedure and would require insurance companies to inform the patient how much their insurance company will pay on this procedure. Employers would be required to offer a choice of insurance plans, with patients having the freedom to choose the method of provider payment in their insurance coverage. This plan would be implemented by eliminating required state programs and by advocating tax-deductible employer and employee contributions to health IRA's.

Universal health insurance coverage would assure no person would be denied access to a health care system. The AMA's plan states, "All Americans, regardless of their income, should have insurance to cover their basic health care needs through private insurance or through government financed programs." This would mean that all employers are required to provide health insurance for all workers and their dependents regardless of income or the size of the company. For those who change jobs, coverage would be guaranteed by the new employer without any waiting period or preexisting condition limitations. Tax assistance and limited premiums for small businesses would be provided so the same group coverage as larger companies would be available. Physicians would then be urged to accept insurance payments as payment-in-full for low income patients. AMA also suggests that by strengthening Medicare funding, the Medicare program for older Americans would be financially secure well into the next century.

The AMA plan suggests that quality assurance encourages physicians to provide the best medical information to their patients and encourages them to follow the best ethical standards of medicine. It also encourages the patient to adopt a healthy lifestyle. Freedom of choice would allow individuals to choose their physician as well as their preferred method of paying for health care. Health system reform is an enormous challenge and the AMA plan is one to be considered in anticipation that older women may have available to them a more complete health care plan that they can support through private or public assistance.

Another organization, the National Association of Social Workers (NASW), is supporting a single-payer, publicly financed insurance plan for all Americans, titled The National Health Care Act of 1992. This plan is defined in a NASW documentary film titled "The Time Has Come." The National Association of Social Workers has supported the introduction of this bill in the U.S. Senate by Senator Daniel Inouye of Hawaii. This bill fundamentally restructures our current health care system. Overall, it will be federally administered and the states will be individually responsible for delivery of health services and payment to the providers.

The bill provides universal coverage for high quality and cost-efficient health, mental health, and long term care through a single-payer national health care system. States have the responsibility to ensure delivery of health services, payment to all providers, and planning in accordance with federal guidelines. Enrollees would have the freedom to choose from among a full range of public and private providers, including alternative delivery plans. Private insurance coverage for benefits provided through the national health program would be discontinued. Coverage is extended to all persons residing in the United States. Enrollment takes place in the state of primary residence; portability of benefits extends across states (NASW, 1992).

The National Association of Social Workers' informational film on this proposed National Health Care Act (1992) further explains the suggested health care plan. Covered benefits through the plan would be extensive and address the needs of the aging women as well as others. The plan promotes preventive care and adds new health education and health promotion services through a variety of community-based settings. Care coordination will be stressed in primary care and is the point of entry for long-term care.

With this plan, a new federal agency is to be established to administer the health care program, with policy direction provided by a national health care advisory board representing health care experts and consumers. Many programs that are independent today would be folded into the program, and individual states would be required to administer the programs in accordance with federal guidelines. The advisory board and some less formal advocate organizations will ensure the implementation of the health care program. The benefits will be accessed to assure fully' funded health care for all: expanded comprehensive benefits including long term and home and community based care; mental health services covered the same as other health care benefits; freedom to choose own provider; and, elimination of current patchwork of public and private insurers.

The program is to be financed primarily through a federal dedicated tax on personal income and through corporate taxes. Additional sources of revenue include state and federal contributions that approximate the government's current health expenditures and increases in cigarette and alcohol taxes. Hospitals would receive global budgets for operating costs and the purchase of high-tech equipment would be regulated by the state. All tax increases are earmarked for health care and all revenues are to be placed in a national health care trust fund. Negotiated fee schedules for all practitioners including doctors, nurses, social workers and other professionals would be set and administered through the states. NASW policy developers presume most individuals would pay less, or near the same amount, through the tax system for expanded benefits than what they are currently paying through premiums and other out-of-pocket costs. "Health care under this plan would no longer be a privilege but a right for everyone," the NASW film, "The Time Has Come" (1992) concludes.

Gilbert and Gilbert (1989), when addressing the fundamental issues in health care, agree they relate to cost containment, quality, and access. With increasing pressures for universal health care entitlement, unprecedented increases in health care expenditures, and a continually growing need, e.g., in response to sociomedical problems such as an expanding aging population, cost containment stands as the overriding priority. The key question to be resolved is how the health care cost burden can be lightened or redistributed, while maintaining quality and extending access.

The plans outlined above are two possible options to be considered in answer to the health care crisis. There may be many other programs or proposed legislation on the drawing boards. Some suggest it would be wise for the administration to review present tax codes regarding medical expenses. Presently, the tax code allows Americans to deduct only that portion of medical expenses that exceed 7.5% of the adjusted gross income. For many who are older or live at the poverty level (currently about $15,000 per year), medical expenses must exceed approximately $1,125 before they can deduct a penny. Would it not be wise to look at the option that taxpayers be permitted to deduct 100% of their medical expenses (Salt Lake Tribune, 1992)? Older women living on set incomes would find this option one which would certainly assist them if health care expenses continue to be an individual responsibility. Those who have an adequate income, although it may be near the poverty level, would also find this beneficial if they are going to continue to be responsible for part of their health care expenses.

It is clear that there will be changes in health policy within the next few years. These anticipated changes could make major health delivery systems much more responsive to the special population of older women but only if older women are about to become more involved, not only in their own health care, but in the policies which govern how that health care is delivered.

HEALTH CARE TREATMENT

What do women expect their health care should include? When taking a small survey of ten women over 65 years and ten women under 65 years, but over 55, whose health was identified as good, the twenty responded as to their health care needs in this manner: eight women, five over 65 and three under 65, said their health care should include care for all health needs they may have; two over 65 and three under 65 thought their health care should include what they could afford to pay for, and each added that they were anticipating having no serious health needs in the future. None of the respondents had a special health insurance plan for extended day care, long-term care or nursing home care. They each expected Medicare and Medicaid to finance any health care they may need.

Four individuals under 65 said they hoped, but did not know if they could expect to have health care for any serious illnesses that they may have. Examples named by them were Alzheimer's disease, cancer, heart attacks, heart trouble, pneumonia, and one mentioned the HIV virus. This small survey seemed to indicate that many women, if this twenty is a representative sample of healthy older women, have thought about their health care in the future but have not identified a plan which would care for them in case of a serious disabling illness or accident.

Only five women among these twenty surveyed mentioned financing health care if needed, although it is common knowledge that health care is an expensive item in today's society. Women are especially likely to lack health care insurance because so many of them are low-wage workers in jobs that do not provide medical coverage. Indeed, being married is a better predictor of health insurance coverage for women than is their employment. The fact that proportionately fewer women are married today has increased their vulnerability (Arendell, 1988). Further, discrimination patterns in the broader society continue to influence power transactions. Rosebeth Kanter's extended discussion of problems that women encounter in large organizations suggests that they are often excluded from decision making because of gender-based prejudice and because they lack access to old-boy networks (Kanter, 1977). Experience in decision making roles certainly does not prepare women to take leadership roles as they become older and this is reflected in how they view the financing of health care as well as planning appropriately for their own health care needs.

Prejudice often prompts people to favor relatively punitive or restrictive policies toward the members of specific groups. Widespread and pervasive prejudice is often called institutional prejudice, which refers to those overt or covert policies that systematically restrict or discriminate against the members of a specific group (Jansson, 1990). Older women who demand health care attention are often discriminated against as a group. They are classified in some medical settings as always having something physical wrong with them, always demanding more care than is necessary, and in some medical settings individuals are not interested in caring for the aging as they can do little to improve the quality of their lives. An example of this is the most recent model proposed for resolving the national health care crises in the state of Oregon. The plan concentrates on preventive medicine, such as maternity care, while giving a much lower priority to high-risk, expensive treatments aimed at prolonging the lives of the terminally ill or the elderly. The arguments and questions of such a plan center around what is the probability that treatment will save a life, and to what degree does treatment allow a person to return to their former healthy state. Many in the state of Oregon and throughout the country have lobbied against such a plan because it would discriminate against specific groups as the older population, the disabled and persons with irreversible health problems.

These discriminatory health issues should force individual groups, such as groups representing older women, to take their health care into their own hands. Some older women have sought health care from those whose main practice is in gerontology. This segment of professionals looks at aging as one of the developmental stages of life and thus looks for ways and means to support this phase and provide a quality of life that is present and possible for such a phase.

The percentage of medically trained individuals, specifically in gerontology, has always been low, although many of the medical specialties address aging problems such as arthritis, heart disease, liver and gall bladder, Alzheimer's disease, etc. Older persons have been satisfied with this segmented form of health care in the past, but because of the continual rise in health care costs, we may see a decided change in the next few years in these medical specialties. As more and more women are admitted to medical school, we are seeing groups of women not only interested in medical practice with women but with older women specifically. There has been a development in many communities throughout the United States of Women's Centers within hospital settings. These Women's Centers focus their treatment and research around all phases of women's lives from early years, usually early teens, to the older women, including those far beyond 65. This innovative way of treating women's health problems has assisted in not only creating a setting where health care problems are addressed by professionals who are trained to address women's health needs, but these professionals are specifically interested in women of all ages and have a goal of addressing the older women's population as their practice specialty. These new centers within hospital settings have found that the maternity needs of women are only one phase of women's lives where health care is an important issue. Through professional research, new programs to address the health needs of older women have become a prominent part of the care delivered in the Women's Centers.

Many believe that in the later stages of life older women are devalued by society on account of both their age and gender, and hence are likely to be impoverished and vulnerable as they approach death. Although women live longer today, they can expect increased and longer periods of chronic health problems. Women tend to have more chronic diseases and disabilities than men, partly because of their greater longevity (Schneider & Guralnik, 1990). Public policies of today do not seem to support or allow changes which assist women to become older with grace.

Health care organizations must become impactful to make public policy changes that will address the needs of older women. A current example of an organization trying to do this is Hospice. This organization assists those who need care during the final years of their life. In England, where this organization was founded over ten years ago, there are now in operation over 25 hospices for the dying. In the United States there are only a few in existence, but many groups are actively organizing and planning to open hospices to provide comforts and care to the dying and their families that cannot easily be offered in a large hospital. The U.S. movement has been bogged down partly due to technical obstacles, including policy related to questions like whether private insurers and Medicaid will cover hospice care, and licensing regulations. There are also philosophical questions involved. Hospices are based on doctors and patients admitting the truth about an illness, and it is debated whether either group is truly willing to do so. One ardent hospice advocate who thinks they should is Dr. Josephine Magno, a cancer specialist at Georgetown Medical Center. "When you stop treating, you are admitting failure," she points out. "It is easier to go on treating than to admit failure. But that is why the hospice concept is such a great thing, because it allows the physician to say, 'Okay, we cannot cure you any more, but we can start caring for you'" (Eron, 1979). Perhaps this is a concept which should be adopted by groups supporting health care for older women.

It appears few women want something different than any older person. Older women have some definite health needs which differ from older men, so when organizations like the American Association of Retired Persons (AARP) and other advocate groups for aging individuals march on Capital Hill for changes in health care legislation, they should include a strong representation from older women since they are the group within that population that has the most to lose under the health care policies of today.

Another organization supporting changes in health care legislation for a specific population is the Alzheimer's Association. Eleven years ago, relatively few Americans had even heard of Alzheimer's disease. Yet, today, this progressive, irreversible brain disease is recognized as one of the most devastating maladies of our time. And, unfortunately, our future (Fasano, 1986). It is a known fact that over forty-three percent of all Americans who turn 65 this year will eventually enter a nursing home, and many of these have Alzheimer's disease. Twenty-five percent of that group will stay at least one year at a cost of $30,000 to $40,000. The Long-Term Care Family Security Act introduced in the spring of 1992 pledges to make long-term care part of health care reform no matter what form is to be considered for adoption (Alzheimer's Association Newsletter, 1992).

It is estimated four million Americans are currently affected with Alzheimer's disease which is estimated to snowball to 14 million by the middle of the next century. Alzheimer's disease costs America over $90 billion a year, with many individuals paying through a cruel game of Russian roulette. If they are unlucky, they'll get stuck with a bill they cannot afford. We need to lower this risk, making long-term care affordable for everyone. The caregivers of the elderly are at greater risk. One in three caregivers are over 65 years-old and 40% of caregivers are husbands at least 75 years-old or older. This places women at an even greater risk since research shows that Alzheimer's disease is two to three times more common in women than in men (Fasano, 1986). Medicaid for Alzheimer's patients is available only after a family spends almost all the money they have on long-term care. Even as families approach poverty, in a growing number of states they can get no help (Alzheimer's Association Newsletter, 1992). The Alzheimer's Association is now engaged in a nationwide effort to educate the public, opinion leaders, and policy makers about long-term care. The Association is recommending to Congress that any long-term care insurance policies being sold must not exclude or limit benefits based on Alzheimer's disease.

As the over 65 population continues to grow at a steady pace, so does the demand for long-term care services. How to provide and pay for such services are crucial issues facing lawmakers today. In the future the long-term care debate on Capitol Hill must be part of the discussion on health care reform. Choices of services for older women who will experience needs for health care during their advanced years must be different than they are today.

FUTURE CHANGES IN HEALTH CARE

While speculating about the future direction of health policy, it is appropriate to examine some of the factors which will determine the demand for changes in health care. These should include older women's needs and concerns; what groups may be new and impactful in the legislative process, and who is to take the leadership role in making these changes in health care.

Women must assert their special concerns and take action to control their health care and improve their health. Healthy practices throughout life including the later years, can have a significant positive impact on the quality of life. The American Association of Retired Persons (1988) developed suggestions to improve women's health care. The improvement of women's health care, no matter what their financial or social status, was defined as meaning taking action through prevention, detection, and treatment. Preventive actions include: (1) eating right through sufficient intake of calcium and fiber, and limiting intake of fat and sodium; (2) getting exercise through finding a form of exercise that meets one's physical abilities, such as walking in the neighborhood, joining a fitness club or class, and looking for senior swim activities; (3) quitting smoking, first through changing to a brand lower in tar and nicotine and reducing the number of cigarettes smoked and then to joining a support group to kick the habit for good; and (4) keeping a healthy frame of mind through group participation, making regular visits to a community center, taking a class, volunteering, maintaining friendships and reaching out to other women. Detection actions include an annual check-up and screening for blood pressure, cholesterol levels, colon cancer, breast cancer, and uterine cancer. Of special importance to older women is the ability to use the health care effectively: acting as a wise and assertive consumer of health care in finding out about services available through Medicare/Medicaid; getting a second opinion if surgery is recommended; and expressing needs to one's doctor and insisting that he or she listen. Many predict that when older women consider themselves the active consumers of health care and health options they will find power to make change on how health services are delivered.

Health research must continue in all aspects of health care to assist us to combat the more common diseases and health problems for those who continue to live longer each year. Research is also needed for diseases like Alzheimer's, about which we know little except what we see, yet we know older women more than older men show signs of the disease. Support must be found to continue research which may find the cause of this devastating disease. Research to assist women as they become older to find ways to sustain and continue their independence is important so this population is not one who becomes more of a strain on the resources of society. And continued research is needed into the development stages of women with specific emphasis on the needs of older women.

Beyond women participating in their own health care and health care choices, and continued research to assist us to know the latest on health issues, who can the nation count on to take the lead in changing public policy related to health care? The elections of the '90s may have placed a group in power who will understand this need and be willing to take some action. Women historically have been missing from the halls of the U.S. Congress. Up until the '90s only 6% of the representatives and just 2% of the senators were women. These statistics should and did anger women, especially the older women who have had many years of experience with the political process. One group who set out to change that picture and the hope of women of today to become part of the decision making bodies of this country is a group named EMILY'S List. This group through financial support has assisted a newly elected body of women to appear in Washington, D.C. in January 1993. It is anticipated that this new group of elected women will change the picture for all women.

EMILY'S List is one worth noting, as this type of women's organized power can be transferable into organizing after elections as well as before. Twelve years ago, Ellen Malcolm founded the Wisdom Fund and used the power of her own money to fund programs for women and minorities which would prepare them for political positions. Ms. Malcolm, next in 1984, with a handful of women from the National Women's Political Caucus started EMILY'S List. EMILY'S List exists to invest in campaigns of Democratic women candidates and to get them elected to political positions in Washington, D.C. where they can represent and control legislation with their main focus on women. EMILY'S List supported only women of the Democratic party. The challenge is now to get women of all parties to organize in the same manner, developing an opportunity for financial support to any woman who wishes to work toward infiltrating the old boy network of the national political scene. These types of organizations will take women's stories to Washington and work toward changes for women. For the first year in history, 47 women will be representing their states in the U.S. House of Representatives and 6 women will be representing their state as members of the United States Senate. Although these women will undoubtedly participate in all policy issues, when it comes to health care and older women, they will be most sensitive to the needs and the lack of appropriate health care options for this special population.

Another advantage for women will be that the efforts of this new group of women on the national level will model the value of women in politics, thus encouraging talented women interested in making a change in public policy to also run for political offices. We should be able to anticipate as we move into the 21st century that over half of those acting on public policy decisions will be women coming to office with great concern for all women. The horizon is brightening and older women will certainly be the beneficiaries of that new dawn.

REFERENCES

Abramovitz, Mimi (1987) "Privatizing Health Care: The Bottom Line Is Society Loses," *The Nation,* Oct. 17, 410-412.

Abramovitz, Mimi (1988) *Regulating The Lives of Women: Social Policy From Colonial Times to the Present,* Boston, Massachusetts, South End Press.

Allsop, J. (1989) "Health," *The New Politics of Welfare: An Agenda for the 1990's?* Ed. by M. McCarthy, 53-81.

Alzheimer's Association Newsletter, 1992, 12-3.

American Medical Association, (1992) "Health Access America," AMA Brochure, AM18:92-429(C):5M:8/92.

American Association of Retired Persons (1988) *Action for a Healthier Life: A Guide for Mid-Life and Older Women,* AARP, Washington, D.C., #D13474.

Arendell, Teresa (1988) "Unmarried Women in a Patriarchal Society: Impoverishment and Access to Health Care Across the Life Cycle," *Poverty and Social Welfare in the United States,* Ed. Donald Tomaskovic-Devey, Boulder, Colorado, Westview Press, 53-81.

Committee on a National Research Agenda on Aging (1991) *Extending Life, Enhancing Life: A National Research Agenda on Aging,* Ed. E.T. Lonergan, Washington, D.C., National Academy Press.

Corder, L.S. and Manton, K.G. (1991) "National Surveys and the Health and Functioning of the Elderly: The Effects of Design and Content," *Journal of the American Statistical Association,* 86, 513-525.

DiNitto, D. (1991) *Social Welfare: Politics and Public Policy,* 3rd Ed. New Jersey, Prentice Hall, Inc.

Eron, C. (1979) "Women in Medicine & Health Care," *The Book of Records and Achievements,* New York, Anchor Press, 197-233.

Fasano, M.A. (1986) *Creative Care for the Person with Alzheimer's,* New Jersey, Brady Book, Prentice Hall, Inc.

Gilbert, N. and Gilbert B. (1989) *The Enabling State, Modern Welfare Capitalism in America,* New York, Oxford University Press.

Guralnik, J.M. and Kaplan, G.A. (1989) "Predictors of Healthy Aging: Prospective Evidence from the Alameda County Study," *America Journal of Public Health,* 75, 127-128.

Holden, K.C. (1988) "Poverty and Living Arrangements Among Older Women: Are Changes in the Well-Being of Elderly Women Understood?" *Journal of Gerontology,* 43, 22-27.

Holden, K.C. (1989) "Women's Economic Status in Old Age and Widowhood," *Women's Life Cycle & Economic Insecurity, Problems & Proposals,* Ed. by M. N. Ozawa, New York, Praeger, 143-165.

Jansson, B.S. (1990) *Social Welfare Policy, From Theory to Practice,* California, Wadsworth Publishing Co.

Kane, R.L., Ouslander, J.G. and Abrass, I.B. (1989) *Essentials of Clinical Geriatrics,* 2nd Edition, New York, McGraw-Hill.

Kanter, R. (1977) *Men and Women of the Corporation,* New York, Basic Books.

Karger, H.J. and Stoesz, D. (1990) "The American Health Care System," *American Social Welfare Policy, A Structural Approach,* New York, Longman, 192-214.

Light, E. and Lebowitz, B.D. (1989) *Alzheimer's Disease Treatment and Family Stress: Directions for Research,* Rockville, Maryland, National Institute of Mental Health.

Martin, G.T., Jr. (1990) "Health," *Social Policy in the Welfare State,* New Jersey, Prentice Hall, 123-157.

National Association of Social Workers (1992) "The Time Has Come," National Health Care Video Tape, Produced by NASW, Washington, D.C.

Rice, D.P. (1989) "Long-Term Care for the Elderly," *Women's Life Cycle & Economic Insecurity, Problems & Proposals,* Ed. by M.N. Ozawa, New York, Praeger, 170-190.

Salt Lake Tribune, November 10, 1992.

Schneider, E.L. and Guralnik, J.M. (1990) "The Aging of America: Impact on Health Care Costs," *Journal of the American Medical Association,* 263, 2335-2340.

Suzman, R. and Riley, M.W. (1985) "Introducing the 'Oldest Old,'" *Milbank Memorial Fund Quarterly,* 63, 177-186.

Taeuber, C.M. (1991) "Profile of Americans Elderly," Census Bureau Report, Washington, D.C.

Trattner, Walter I. (1989) *From Poor Law to Welfare State, A History of Social Welfare in America,* 4th Ed., New York, Free Press.

U.S. Bureau of the Census (1984) "Projections of the Population of the United States, 1983-2080," *Current Population Reports,* Series P-25, #952, Washington, D.C., U.S. Government Printing Office.

U.S. Bureau of the Census (1986) Statistical Abstract of the United States, Washington, D.C., U.S. Government Printing Office, 96-99.

U.S. Bureau of the Census (1987) Statistical Abstract of the United States, Washington, D.C., U.S. Government Printing Office, 84-88.

U.S. Department of Health and Human Services (1987) Social Security Bulletin: Annual Statistical Supplement, Washington, D.C., U.S. Government Printing Office, 75-76.

Women and Healthy Aging: Conclusion

Alice A. Young, PhD
J. Dianne Garner, DSW

In the early morning hours
She gropes her way through darkness.
Slow shuffling feet and the thump of her walker
Break the sound of silence.
Gnarled hands reach for the lamp
Casting shadows on faded wallpaper.
She lowers herself cautiously
Wincing only slightly.
Her gray hair flows unchallenged
Attesting to her still free spirit.
Armed with magnifier and glasses
Stiff fingers caress a well-loved book.
Yellowed pages crackle as they turn
Bringing anticipation to a once strong heart.
And in opaque eyes burns a muted fire
As she remembers running through autumns' leaves
and once again reads Whitman.

–J. Dianne Garner

Alice A. Young is Professor and Dean, School of Nursing, and J. Dianne Garner is Professor and Chair, Department of Social Work, Washburn University, Topeka, KS.

[Haworth co-indexing entry note]: "Women and Healthy Aging: Conclusion." Young, Alice A., and J. Dianne Garner. Co-published simultaneously in the *Journal of Women & Aging* (The Haworth Press, Inc.) Vol. 5, No. 3/4, 1993, pp. 221-226; and: *Women and Healthy Aging: Living Productively in Spite of It All* (ed: J. Dianne Garner, and Alice A. Young), The Haworth Press, Inc., 1993, pp. 221-226. Multiple copies of this article/chapter may be purchased from The Haworth Document Delivery Center [1-800-3-HAWORTH; 9:00 a.m.-5:00 p.m. (EST)].

The purpose of this work has been to explore what is known about healthy living among older women, with particular emphasis on overcoming illness and adversity for enjoyment of long, productive, personally fulfilling lives. Several authors have presented helpful medical information for understanding the common illnesses and health problems afflicting women as they grow older and have offered prescriptions for dealing with the various associated complexities of disease, structural changes and functional limitations. Concomitant feelings of powerlessness, low self worth, isolation and depression experienced by aging women with health problems are discussed by several of the authors. Others have explored the demographics of aging, the importance of attitudes and definitions in shaping lives, the problems of discrimination, lack of financing and the inadequacy of health care services for elderly women. The call for health care reform and greater involvement of older American women in shaping public policy is loud and clear. The authors of this work have offered suggestions for coping with illness and loss, but most importantly, they have provided models for healthy living–by the example of their own lives and by illustrations of people they have known. This work can serve as a kind of handbook, not merely of "survival" techniques, but of strategies for maintaining positive attitudes and healthy lifestyles while aging.

Common themes have emerged from the works presented here. How one defines "health" is critical in shaping one's response to health problems–illness, adversity or limitations. Health, most authors agree, is more than the absence of illness. Of the multiple changes that accompany the aging process, some are more troublesome than others. Some are physiological processes that occur normally in the course of aging (menopause, structural and sensory alterations). Some are diseases that require medical treatment (heart disease, cancer, diabetes). Some are conditions, syndromes or illnesses that do not have identified causation, known cures, or even satisfactory treatment programs which are effective in reducing painful and annoying symptoms (sensory loss, arthritis, Alzheimer's disease, cancer, osteoporosis).

Burnside differentiates between disease (a condition that impairs performance) and illness (individuals' perceptions and behaviors in response to the disease and the impact it has on their lives). Since no one is completely healthy, even in youth, it is imperative that the responses learned for coping with illness throughout life are effective for dealing with the higher incidence of illness that increases as one moves into the later years. "To be the best one can be" is a goal for elderly women presented by the authors of this work. Sometimes that means facing the reality of aging head on and not denying the aches and pains, nor diminishing the reality of impairment or disease when it occurs. Sometimes it means redefining oneself as an older person, developing a new sense of self-appreciation, "connectedness" and purpose in life, while legitimizing the inherent freedoms within and providing new opportunities for their creative release (Burnside, Roberto, Peden, Newman, Souder, Kinderknecht, Garner).

Guthrie, Rimmer, Lord and others stress the importance of recognizing the changes that do occur in disease processes, doing what you can about them, whether it is seeking factual information, getting a cane to assist with ambulation or a hearing aid for better communication, undergoing medical treatment or surgery, changing one's life style as necessary and, most importantly, developing a positive attitude, so that "in spite of it all," you can get on with living. The importance of personal attitudes for experiencing quality of life is a theme that resounds from many authors here (Burnside, Lord, Newman, Garner, Kinderknecht).

Even as physical disabilities engender restrictions in body movements and inflict limitations in some respects, living with illness can be a "freeing" experience in other dimensions. When coping strategies used in the past to deal with adversity are no longer effective, a person needs to find new and different ways of living. Out of conflicts, pain, suffering and limitation, there can emerge new strengths of the person that outweigh the temptations toward futility and hopelessness. With the right attitudes, illness can be a transforming experience. The richness of one's past life experiences can provide the wisdom and resources necessary for embracing the present condition as yet another opportunity for growth and enrichment. Several of the authors here describe the deepening spirituality, new appreciations and insights, and the creativity that emerges when elderly women choose life rather than illness as their focal point. Ruth Harriet Jacobs' poetry throughout this volume is a living example.

How attitudes of society and social policy affect the quality of life and health care for older women is described graphically by Jorgensen and Belgrave. Problems of poverty and poor health care for elderly women is a growing concern as increasing numbers of women find themselves today living alone, with more chronic health problems and without adequate finances or third party coverage. How to provide and pay for long term care for the elderly with conditions such as Alzheimer's and other debilitating diseases is a critical issue facing us today. Jorgensen calls for the elimination of discriminatory health coverage, whether gender or condition based, as a primary step in the larger arena of health care reform. The call for health care reform is coming from all avenues today, consumers, elderly advocacy lobbying groups such as AARP and the Gray Panthers, and from the providers themselves. Jorgensen describes the efforts of the American Medical Association (AMA) and the National Association of Social Workers (NASW) in developing proposals for health care reform. In addition, the American Nurses' Association (ANA) has developed its *Agenda for Health Care Reform*, signed on by many other professional organizations. What all these proposals have in common is the premise that health care is a basic human right and problems of universal access to services, cost control and quality assurance must be addressed.

Jorgensen challenges older women themselves to adopt a more healthy lifestyle which embraces nutrition, exercise, a positive attitude and use of preventive screenings. Rimmer, Lord, Newman, Peden and Richards describe many of the very real problems of elderly women who do take advantage of available primary health care for screenings for heart disease and cancer. Detection programs are not adequate for diagnosing many cancers in the early stages and many women's heart conditions are not as readily detected as men's because the mechanisms for detection and the norms have all been developed for the male population. The medical community has yet to understand differences in diagnosis, treatment and prognosis of women's heart problems or how risk factors may vary for men and women. Belgrave and others highlight the age and gender bias that is prevalent in health care delivery today. Older patients do not receive the same care as younger patients and women are often discriminated against in access to services, types of services received and in length and quality of their treatment.

There are many unanswered questions about the differential health care for women and men. Traditionally, it has been thought to be more socially acceptable for women to seek health services than for men to do so, which may explain the greater utilization of preventive health services into older age by women than men. But it does not explain why women tend to have greater incidence of and more limitations from chronic health problems than men or why men receive more procedures (Belgrave) or why women are less likely than men to be referred for cardiac catheterizations, angioplasty or coronary bypass surgery for similar presenting symptoms (Rimmer). Neither does it explain why older women receive less adequate care for breast cancer than younger women or why male medical handling of menopause in women is inadequate and inconsistent (Belgrave, Peden, Newman, Lord, Richards). Roberto discusses the frustrations women experience over inconsistent, conflicting information and confusing medical advice regarding treatment for problems of osteoporosis. Differing expert opinions, controversy and inconclusive evidence on method, length and value of estrogen replacement therapy for control of symptoms are also common experiences of women during menopause.

For the majority of women, life will continue after menopause for another 30 to 40 years. The challenge facing women as they enter the prime mid-years of the 50s is to prepare themselves for the future by becoming informed consumers and by taking an active role in making health care decisions that will affect the quality of their lives. Jorgensen points out that although many women over the age of 55 have given some thought to their health care in the future, few have taken concrete steps to select a plan which addresses and finances their individual needs in event of serious illness, accident or chronic health problems. The need for better education of women regarding their health care is apparent.

Autonomy in decision making promotes a sense of power and self-esteem that elderly women need in order to maintain their integrity during illness and times of adversity. The maximum health potential for aging women is individually defined and is related to multiple variables, such as type of illness or impairment, degree to which the individual has accepted the condition and been transformed by it, one's education or knowledge about the condition, one's personal resources and coping skills, social support systems available in the form of caregivers, family and friends and the degree of assistance needed.

The role of health care providers in relation to various health problems encountered by elderly women is addressed by several authors in this work. Providers have an important responsibility in facilitating problem solving of elderly women in making their life changes and developing coping skills. Providers can offer assistance in minimizing limitations and maximizing individuals' strengths. They can also help the elderly to reshape their environment to better serve their needs. Peden and Newman highlight women's potential to become their "most memorable self" during the post menopausal period on into the remaining decades propelled with the "new energy surge" that hails the end to the hormonal fluctuations of menopause.

Elderly women today generally have an unchartered course for the future. Few norms are available to them and few examples of what constitutes successful aging are actually explicated. Research is desperately needed on all of the diseases that women commonly experience, the needs of older women, the aging process in women, and successful coping mechanisms for maintaining independence (Jorgensen). This compiled edition points the direction for the work which is yet to be done as it attests to the spirit and resiliency of multiple older women who have successfully met the challenges of living with adversity.

At Eighty

Two years past eighty
I forget a lot of things
I don't want to remember
Like watching my words.
I remember a lot of things
I thought I had forgotten
like Miss Brown
who made kindergarten
another home

Two years past eighty
I spot a new bird
learn a wildflower's name
see a great grandchild smile
hear live, for the first time
Bach's Sonata in C Major,
tell the President off,
drink a new wine,
and make new friends.

–Ruth Harriet Jacobs, PhD
Reprinted with permission
from Knowledge, Ideas & Trends, Inc.

Ruth Harriet Jacobs is Researcher, Wellesley College Center for Research on Women, Wellesley, MA 02181.

[Haworth co-indexing entry note]: "At Eighty." Jacobs, Ruth Harriet. Co-published simultaneously in the *Journal of Women & Aging* (The Haworth Press, Inc.) Vol. 5, No. 3/4, 1993, p. 227; and: *Women and Healthy Aging: Living Productively in Spite of It All* (ed: J. Dianne Garner, and Alice A. Young), The Haworth Press, Inc., 1993, p. 227.

Index

AARP (American Association of Retired Persons), 78, 215,216,224
Absorptiometry in osteoporosis, 47
Accidents. *See* Safety
Acetohexamide (Dymelor), 93
Activity level, 13-14
ADA. *See* American Diabetes Association (ADA)
Adams, R.N., 36
"Adaptation" (poem), 7
Ageism. *See* Discrimination
Age spots, 28-29
Albers, M., 44
Alcohol use
    and blood lipids, 105,113
    and osteoporosis, 45
Alliance for Aging Research, 157-158
Allison, M., 113
Alternative therapies in arthritis, 65
Alzheimer, A., 140
Alzheimer's Association, 149, 215-216
Alzheimer's disease, 12
    causes and classification, 140-141
    diagnosis, 142-144
    epidemiology, 139-140
    and health care costs, 215-216
    prevalence, 3
    resources, 150-151, 215-216
    strategies for maximizing function, 147-150
    symptoms and disease progression, 144-146
    treatment, 146-147
    vs. multi-infarct dementia, 139-140,143

Alzheimer's Disease and Related Disorders Association (ADRDA), 15,142,148
AMA. *See* American Medical Association (AMA)
American Association of Retired Persons. *See* AARP
American Cancer Society, 119,120, 121,122,123,133
American Diabetes Association (ADA), 85,89,94
American Geriatrics Society, 123
American Heart Association, 101, 102,104,106,109
American Medical Association (AMA), 205,224
    "Health Access America" plan, 207-209
American Nurses' Association (ANA), 224
American Psychiatric Association (APA), 139-140
ANA (American Nurses' Association), 224
Anderson, J.J., 68
Anderson, K.O., 74
Angina pectoris, 107-108,113-114. *See also* Heart disease
Angiography, coronary, 108-109,189
Ankylosing spondylitis, 63
Anst, M., 49
Arendell, T., 212
Arthritis
    disease process of, 62-63
    epidemiology, 61-62
    osteo- defined, 62
    physiological impacts, 65-67
    psychosocial impacts, 67-71

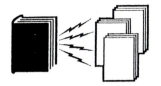

Haworth
DOCUMENT DELIVERY
SERVICE
and Local Photocopying Royalty Payment Form

This new service provides (a) a single-article order form for any article from a Haworth journal and (b) a convenient royalty payment form for local photocopying (not applicable to photocopies intended for resale).

- *Time Saving:* No running around from library to library to find a specific article.
- *Cost Effective:* All costs are kept down to a minimum.
- *Fast Delivery:* Choose from several options, including same-day FAX.
- *No Copyright Hassles:* You will be supplied by the original publisher.
- *Easy Payment:* Choose from several easy payment methods.

Open Accounts Welcome for . . .
- Library Interlibrary Loan Departments
- Library Network/Consortia Wishing to Provide Single-Article Services
- Indexing/Abstracting Services with Single Article Provision Services
- Document Provision Brokers and Freelance Information Service Providers

MAIL or *FAX* THIS ENTIRE ORDER FORM TO:

Attn: **Marianne Arnold**
Haworth Document Delivery Service
The Haworth Press, Inc.
10 Alice Street
Binghamton, NY 13904-1580

or FAX: (607) 722-1424
or CALL: 1-800-3-HAWORTH
(1-800-342-9678; 9am-5pm EST)

PLEASE SEND ME PHOTOCOPIES OF THE FOLLOWING SINGLE ARTICLES:

1) Journal Title: _____
     Vol/Issue/Year:_____Starting & Ending Pages:_____
Article Title:_____

2) Journal Title: _____
     Vol/Issue/Year:_____Starting & Ending Pages:_____
Article Title:_____

3) Journal Title: _____
     Vol/Issue/Year:_____Starting & Ending Pages:_____
Article Title:_____

4) Journal Title: _____
     Vol/Issue/Year:_____Starting & Ending Pages:_____
Article Title:_____

(See other side for Costs and Payment Information)

COSTS: Please figure your cost to order quality copies of an article.

1. Set-up charge per article: $8.00

         ($8.00 × number of separate articles)   _____

2. Photocopying charge for each article:

         1-10 pages: $1.00   _____

         11-19 pages: $3.00   _____

         20-29 pages: $5.00   _____

         30+ pages: $2.00/10 pages   _____

3. Flexicover (optional): $2.00/article   _____

4. Postage & Handling: US: $1.00 for the first article/

         $.50 each additional article   _____

         Federal Express: $25.00   _____

         Outside US: $2.00 for first article/

         $.50 each additional article   _____

5. Same-day FAX service: $.35 per page   _____

6. Local Photocopying Royalty Payment: should you wish to copy the article yourself. Not intended for photocopies made for resale, $1.50 per article per copy (i.e. 10 articles x $1.50 each = $15.00)   _____

          GRAND TOTAL: _____

METHOD OF PAYMENT: (please check one)

❑ Check enclosed   ❑ Please ship and bill. PO # _____

         (sorry we can ship and bill to bookstores only! All others must pre-pay)

❑ Charge to my credit card: ❑ Visa; ❑ MasterCard; ❑ American Express;

Account Number: _____   Expiration date: _____

Signature: *X* _____   Name: _____

Institution: _____   Address: _____

City: _____   State: _____ Zip: _____

Phone Number: _____   FAX Number: _____

MAIL or *FAX* THIS ENTIRE ORDER FORM TO:

Attn: **Marianne Arnold**
Haworth Document Delivery Service
The Haworth Press, Inc.
10 Alice Street
Binghamton, NY 13904-1580

or **FAX:** (607) 722-1424
or **CALL:** 1-800-3-HAWORTH
(1-800-342-9678; 9am-5pm EST)

Date Due